INTIMACY AND DESIRE

How to stimulate a relationship discovering what she/he really wants into the bed. A journey into sexual fantasies in marriage and couples to have good sex and sexual health.

DONNA DARE

© Copyright 2019 - All rights reserved.

The content contained within this book may not be reproduced, duplicated or transmitted without direct written permission from the author or the publisher.

Under no circumstances will any blame or legal responsibility be held against the publisher, or author, for any damages, reparation, or monetary loss due to the information contained within this book. Either directly or indirectly.

Legal Notice:

This book is copyright protected. This book is only for personal use. You cannot amend, distribute, sell, use, quote or paraphrase any part, or the content within this book, without the consent of the author or publisher.

Disclaimer Notice:

Please note the information contained within this document is for educational and entertainment purposes only. All effort has been executed to present accurate, up to date, and reliable, complete information. No warranties of any kind are declared or implied. Readers acknowledge that the author is not engaging in the rendering of legal, financial, medical or professional advice. The content within this book has been derived from various sources. Please consult a licensed professional before attempting any techniques outlined in this book.

By reading this document, the reader agrees that under no circumstances is the author responsible for any losses, direct or indirect, which are incurred as a result of the use of information contained within this document, including, but not limited to, — errors, omissions, or inaccuracies.

Table of Contents

Description 1
Introduction 5
Chapter 1: Different Types of Intimacy 13
Chapter 2: Intimacy and Sex in a Marriage 15
Chapter 3: How to Revive Intimacy 24
   Prioritize Your Relationship 24
   Flirt With Each Other 25
   Create a Habit 25
   Getting In the Mood 26
   Date Nights 26
   Make Them Feel Special 27
   Terms of Endearment 27
   Don't Let Yourself Go 28
   Don't Take Arguments to Bed 29
   Increase Your Physical Contact 29
Chapter 4: Creating Emotional Intimacy with Your Man ... 30
Chapter 5: Spice Things Up In the Sack 35
Chapter 6: Communication Practices 43
Chapter 7: Forgetting About Past Ghosts 61
Chapter 8: Loving Words Heal Relationships 74
   How to Express Love Words 78
   Using Words of Love to Inspire the Relationship - 3 Tips for Men to Learn 80
Chapter 9: What Women Want; What Men Want 83
Chapter 10: Tips to Have More Intimacy in Every Situation 88
Chapter 11: Restoring Intimacy in Your Marriage 96
Chapter 12: Tantric Sex For Marriage 102
   The Yin and the Yang: Which is male and which is female? ... 103
      Shiva and Shakti 104
      Understanding the opposites 104
      My partner is my beloved 105
      The Desire Spectrum 106

You feel empowered to say what you want! 106
Chapter 13: Teachings of tantric sex **108**
- Breathe 108
- Relax 110
- Sounds can help! 112
- Eye contact is essential 115
- Pay attention 116
- Always be present 117

Chapter 14: Understand the Challenges Created by Social Messages **119**
- Challenges for Women 119
  - Distractibility During Sex 119
  - Loss of Sexual Interest as a Mom 120
  - Low Sexual Desire 120
- Challenges for Men 121
  - Midlife Crisis 121
  - Sexual Dysfunction 122
- Challenges for Couples 123
  - Sexless Relationship/Marriage 123
  - Emotional Distance 124
- One Couple's Plight Through the Lens of Social Messages 125

Chapter 15: Romance After The Kids **128**
- Update Each Other Every Week 128
- Sharing the Parenting 129
- Finding Time for Intimacy 130
- Get Yourselves a Babysitter 131
- Pay More Attention To Your Spouse 132
- Appreciation, Admiration and Affection 134

Chapter 16: Improving Intimacy **135**
Chapter 17: More Intimacy in 7 Days **142**
Conclusion **154**

Description

Sexual connection and satisfaction is a key factor to a more fulfilling relationship. Many couples experience a decline of sexual desire and frequency of intercourse over the course of a long-term relationship, but studies have shown that couples who work to keep the passion alive are often happier. By viewing sex as part of the glue that binds you a greater intimacy can be achieved and a closeness that will satisfy your needs can be achieved.

Here we will examine a few key tips to keep your sex life interesting and are facts that all happy couples know are unquestionably true about having a great sex life!

Maybe you are one of those rare couples that have incredible amounts of fantastic sex even years into your relationship, and if you are, well done you, maybe you should write a book and tell everyone your secret!! If not, then read on! It is a true fact that in general the longer a couple has been together the less sex they will be having. Now that is not altogether a bad thing as long as you realize that good sex is important and as long as you are aware of the little things you do that drive your partner crazy with lust and you are still doing them. Maybe think about trying a few new moves, be creative! Providing you have a relationship that allows you to be truthful with each other the skies the limit!

Remembering that as you age and your body changes that you will both need more time to become aroused and climax. Make time for sex, forget the hurried frantic sexual encounters often reminiscent of your early years. Can it really be a bad thing to take more time having intercourse? Think about it, a relaxed interruption free atmosphere, great surroundings and comfortable locations can only improve matters. In fact, by taking more time and introducing new relaxed techniques you can open up all-new experiences. Make sure you take time to show physical affection when having sex. Kissing for long periods of time can lead to heightened emotions and a greater feeling of sharing a physical bond. It is important to feel connected during this most intimate of acts and by avoiding distractions and committing yourself fully this can be achieved.

Honesty plays a huge part in maintaining a healthy sex life. You may feel that by faking an orgasm you are shielding your partner's feelings but you are creating a dangerous precedent. By starting an honest and meaningful conversation about your physical needs, your expectations and dislikes you can open up the door to a deeply satisfying experience for both of you. Avoid criticism and learn how to suggest positive actions rather than focusing on negative issues. Confide in your partner any changes you would like to try, research new positions and sex aids that you would both be comfortable with! Research can be fun, giggling over the wild and wacky range of toys that are out there and can be found on the internet can bring you closer together. Whilst many couples find it hard to talk about sex good communication is essential to healthy relationships.

This guide will focus on the following:

- Different types of intimacy
- Intimacy and sex in a marriage
- How to revive intimacy
- Creating emotional intimacy with your man
- Spice things up in the sack
- Communication practices
- Things to do as a couple
- Loving words heal relationships

- What women want; what men want
- Tips to have more intimacy in every situation
- Restoring intimacy in your marriage
- Tantric sex for marriage
- Teachings of tantric sex
- Understand the challenges created by social messages
- Romance after the kids
- Improving intimacy
- More intimacy in 7 days... AND MORE!!!

Introduction

Experimentation is essential to maintain healthy interest. Compare your love life to your daily diet, for instance, how would you feel if you were served the same meal, at the same time and on the same plate day after day? Bored, right? So, change things up a bit! Sexual positions are a start, often we rely on tried and trusted sexual positions and that is great for the majority of the time but every now and again explore some new moves! As long as you are aware of your own and your partners' limitations physically you can find new ways to increase stimulation. By choosing new positions you can also overcome problems caused by physical limitations.

Understand the different actions that can be classed as foreplay. Often mundane tasks can become the main activity of a normal day, realizing the potential of these everyday activities can be eye-opening. For instance, if your partner decides to take on one of your least favorite household tasks and maybe vacuums the whole house because he knows you hate doing it, then they are trying to make you happy and that can be one of the sexiest things ever!! Foreplay is often overlooked by people in a long-term relationship and this can lead to resentment and disappointment that will eventually lead to problems both in the bedroom and outside.

Foreplay can often start with the basic act of preparing for intimacy. By dressing sexily, maybe lingerie and a slinky nightie, fixing your hair and adding a bit of make-up can all lead to heightened confidence. Confidence is a major boost to your levels of sexiness and can lead to increased ability to take it that bit further when switching things up!

Maybe the man is the traditional leader in the bedroom, imagine how fun it would be to swap those roles over. Always maintaining awareness of the other partner's feelings, change the roles in the boudoir, there is always the potential for surprise when it comes to making out!

Masturbation is often regarded as a solo activity but can be a fantastic foreplay tool. Showing your partner that you are in control of your own sexuality can be a major turn on. Invite them to join in and you can quite often create a mutual sense of satisfaction. Take it slow and steady and you will find that exploring your partner's methods of masturbation and self-pleasuring can give you interesting ideas when it is your turn to give them pleasure! Think of it as a pleasurable insight into what floats your partner's boat!

Exercise is a great way to improve sexual fitness. Often over time our bodies can become less taut and both sexes can benefit from some simple pelvic floor muscle exercises. One simple method that can be used by both men and women is to contract your bladder as if trying to prevent urination. Do this contraction 5 to 10 times a go and at half a dozen different times of the day. By doing so you are exercising the muscles that contract during orgasm. By flexing and toning these muscles you augment the sensations and make it easier to achieve a satisfying orgasm.

These exercises also tighten the vaginal muscles and increase the flow of blood to the pelvic area meaning that both partners will enjoy a more intense and pleasurable experience during sex.

Whilst they were originally developed to aid relief for people who had given birth or had been involved in accidents it is widely believed that by practicing these simple exercises you can improve not only your sex life but the general control over bladder and bowel. The pelvic floor is also known as your pelvic diaphragm and by increasing the amount of time tightening up these muscles a marked difference in all areas associated with the area should be evident. It is worth pointing out that whilst the exercises replicate the action of stopping urine mid-flow it is actually very dangerous to do so whilst urinating.

A great way to perk up your libido is by removing household objects from your bedroom. It can be distracting to find yourself looking at the picture of granddad on the nightstand, work clothes scattered about the room can just make you think about work-related stuff. Make your bedroom a retreat, use soft colors and materials, think sexy boudoir rather than working bedroom and your mind, and body will respond to these extra stimuli.

Ditch the TV! In the bedroom especially how many of us have fallen asleep to the dulcet tones of some late-night presenter when really, we would love to be falling asleep exhausted by our love lives? Move the goggle box into the den and take time out to talk to each other before sleep. The good old make-out session can soon be replacing mind-numbing TV watching. If that is working for you why not try the same trick in the lounge? If you are not brave enough to ditch it completely the at least set a schedule to turn it off on certain nights.

Don't ignore problems. Whilst erectile dysfunction is a common sexual problem and affects a number of men much less is known about women's problems and how to treat them. Later in life, many women experience vaginal dryness and pain due to lack of lubrication. If lubrication is needed there are many forms of artificial alternatives to choose from. Good old KY jelly can make intercourse a pleasure again. Why not try to make an application a form of foreplay? Often a woman can be too embarrassed to address this condition as it often occurs at the same time as menopause and can lead to feelings of uselessness and somehow feeling less womanly.

A thoughtful and loving partner will be able to take a potentially distressing situation and use it to restore a feeling of sexiness in his partner. Make sure you lubricate slowly and sensually and you will both derive pleasure from the sensations you will arouse. Done correctly this will lead to pain-free and very slippery sex, now who doesn't want that??

The best sex is achieved by taking on board your partner's feelings, fears and hopes and by being the best that you can be you will work together and achieve the ultimate goal, love intimacy and satisfaction.

Recapitulating, intimacy issues are not just intimacy issues. As the sexual activity is a basic instance for pleasure-seeking, whatever happens in it works as a symptom of something else, more general and profound, related to the way we pursue what we want in life. One does not fail at sex, one *also* fails at sex. Why also there? Because it works as the ultimate and key surface where our unconscious self can express itself. Quite often, we do not realize (or deny) what we are passing through until we feel some discomfort or frustration in our sexual life that makes us ask ourselves about it.

In other words, we cannot lie to ourselves in bed as we may do it in other aspects of our lives. We may lie to our partner, but definitely not to ourselves. As long as sex and intimacy are such particular experiences for every person and couple, there is no universal rule to identify if you are failing at it or not. So, the best way to know it is to determine it yourself. Additionally, 'failing' is not a good word to describe intimacy issues.

There is nothing a goal to reach but to find what gives you and your partner pleasure.

Just be extremely honest with you: Do you enjoy your sexual life? Do you feel confident with your partner? Do you have as much sex as you want? Do you reach orgasms with your partner? Do you feel that you would prefer to be with someone else? Do you feel your sexual activity is satisfactory to yourself? Do you want to do something you have never done before but you are not sure about how your partner will react?

Ask yourself these questions and others. Try to find what really separates you from the place you would want to be. As 'failing' is an inaccurate word to talk about sex and intimacy, the same happens with the idea of 'fault'.

Sexuality is something shared, and (in principle) develops in the context of a couple. Nothing means anything without its context, and what could be good for a couple will not for another one. In the same sense, things only happen in their specific coordinates, and would not be possible in other scenarios. What we mean is that if something happens in the sexual life of a couple it will be both people's business. The responsibility is shared as well. Even if whatever happens seems to affect just one person, both should take it as a serious issue that needs to be discussed.

Chapter 1: Different Types of Intimacy

You might be surprised, but there are different types of intimacy in relationships. The two primary types of intimacy are physical and emotional. Because of this, different partners are likely to see different types of intimacy as more important. You and your partner might have two different ideas of what intimacy should look like in your relationship, so it is important that you learn to communicate with these types of things.

Physical intimacy is an intimacy that is shown through physical touch. People who are more interested in physical intimacy tend to feel more connected to their partner through touch. The touch can be non-sexual such as hand-holding, a hand on the shoulder, hugging, and even sitting next to each other with body parts touching. Or, it can be sexual. When you want to turn someone on who is more interested in physical intimacy, you need to use this to your advantage. Use sensual touching of various areas of the body as an opportunity to turn them on.

Emotional intimacy is an intimacy that is given and received through feelings. People who are more interested in emotional intimacy are turned on through words and other things that evoke emotions. They may be more likely to respond to surprises, storytelling, gifts, and more.

Most relationships rely on both types of intimacy, though the balance will be unique to each individual relationship. Finding the perfect balance will require communication and practice as you both learn how to physically and emotionally communicate with each other in a way that nurtures your relationship.

Chapter 2: Intimacy and Sex in a Marriage

Sex in marriage enhances the bond between two partners. It should form part of how two partners interact and express their love for each other. The common belief is that humans might find it hard to mate for life. That is not the case; there are innovative ways to make sex interesting so that partners enjoy each other for life. Some creativity reignites the spark in bed leaving your partner yearning for you every time. Choose to believe that it is not difficult to make sex seem new every time. The right attitude makes sex as interesting as if was the first time.

Sex is as much mental as it is physical. Partners should share a deep connection so that they are always in sync in any activity they carry out together. Sex is one element that requires this sort of connection for it to be totally fulfilling. A sexless marriage is a major problem in many marriages. One spouse may be desperately yearning for touch and physical closeness and when these needs are ignored a major disconnect happens. The spouse may feel unwanted, unappreciated and the couple even stops spending time together. Eye contact lessens and the bond between them weakens and puts the marriage in a risky position. This chapter will focus on the frequently asked questions about sex in marriage and how to deal with them.

The most common question asked about sex is whether it is possible to keep sex interesting after being with your partner for such a long time. Well, it is very possible. There are different ways to ensure that sex remains part of a married couple's life that they always look forward to. It takes a little effort but it is worthwhile since you are with your partner for a lifetime. All it takes is a little cuddling, some new sex positions, love notes, and other simple techniques.

Seduction in marriage can still remain as tantalizing as ever. Sure, it may change with time but it can still be erotic. Partners may explore their sexuality by wearing sexy outfits for each other; especially for women. Even though people have been together for a long time, they should not give up on pleasing their partners. Sexual banter works wonders to rekindle those sexual desires. A woman can decide to visit a sex shop and choose from a wide variety of items they are comfortable with like crotch-less panties, lingerie and feminine wear that is revealing and provokes sexual tension in men. Men are visual creatures and seducing a man may need something like this. Such aspects make sex life wild and more interesting. Partners should look into ways of bringing new experiences into the sex life.

The difficulty with seduction is when two partners have different fetishes. Most couples complain of their partners taking fetishes too far. Some partners hurt each other to derive satisfaction. It has taken a toll on a lot of couples. The reasonable thing to do is to discuss with their partners and even consider the possibility of seeing a therapist. A woman once complained of her sex life with her husband deteriorating over the course of the marriage. It reached a point where the husband would slap her painfully on the face. Such a case demonstrates the way fetishes can be taken too far. Another case is where a man complained of the wife insisting on giving him a prostate massage. The man was very adamant and it formed a basis for argument and disagreement. Seduction and sex should be done under mutual consent, willingness and trust. It does not have to make your partner feel uncomfortable.

The other most commonly asked question about sex in marriage is about erectile dysfunction. Such an issue weighs down sexual energy in a marriage. Erectile dysfunction is a major cause of unhappiness in so many marriages. Sometimes, a woman may feel unattractive and the man may feel a lot of pressure by not being able to satisfy his wife. If the man is not suffering from any medical condition that predisposes them to erectile dysfunction, most of the times it is usually psychological. Medical conditions that predispose one to erectile dysfunction include diabetes. Other habits also cause erectile dysfunction like smoking and inactivity. Men should watch their cholesterol levels.

Erectile dysfunction caused by anxiety can be addressed by communication. The man has to feel the burden of pressure lifted off his chest. A therapist could help in opening up the bottled up feelings so that the man feels comfortable discussing it. Performance anxiety is a major cause of erectile dysfunction. Men with erectile dysfunction often ignore their wives and don't want to have sex which may aggravate tension in the marriage. Marriage counselors also handle a lot of cases like this. For a marriage to move on from this, communication between the partners has to be open and always at its best. Though it may take time, most couples regain their sexual vigor when psychological issues are out of the way. At a later age, women suffer reduced vaginal lubrication and reduced muscle spasms during an orgasm. Such physical hindrances can be addressed by using lubricants and estrogen replacement therapy.

Communication also helps when sex drives differ. In some marriages, sex drive is at different levels where partners are out of sync and may feel disconnected. The only way to solve this is to communicate and talk about their expectations and reason that could be affecting their libido. Sometimes, it could be work-related, family-related or so on. Couples often forget to be thankful for their strong points and choose to focus on how little sex they have in a month rather than just speaking their minds out. Talking about such issues brings synchrony where it could be lacking. As long as the minds are in sync, there will be a middle ground that will be found in sexual matters. As mentioned, even erectile dysfunction can be addressed by simply communicating.

The other commonly asked question about sex is whether exercise helps. Exercise is a major booster of a married couple's sex life. Exercise improves the overall fitness of the body and makes you more attractive. It also improves one confidence which is a major component to pleasing your partner in bed. Through exercise, people acquire endurance and energy to have sex. It sends a variety of 'feel-good hormones' throughout the body which implies a positive effect even to their partners. The effort put into exercise also makes your partner desire you more and appreciate your dedication to staying attractive for them.

Concern about the monotony of sex arises in most couples who have been married for a long time. Sex does not have to be monotonous in marriage. There are a lot of sex advice books both online and in book stores. It helps to read such books some times. Setting the mood for sex is also one way to break the monotony. Setting the mood should be done way in advance before having sex. It can be done by sending texts throughout the day to each other or starting foreplay before you even get into bed and so on. Ignoring your spouse throughout the day is one way to kill the mood. Communication helps keep the flame alive and yields positive lovemaking at the end of the day.

Often, couples compare their sex lives with others. The issue of sex should be private and should not be compared. Couples often forget that sex cannot be perfect every time as portrayed in movies or as friends would put it. Sometimes, it has its imperfection which is quite normal. To maintain the eagerness between each other, couples can try to abstain and build up desire for each other. It is the little things that make sex more interesting. Trying to look for perfect sex is futile and partners have to understand each other every time. For example, an issue that affects men psychologically is penis size. Many men sometimes feel inadequate about the size of their penis. Truthfully, it's all in the mind. When men worry too much about their penis size it can even likely cause erectile dysfunction. It is not just about the size of the penis but it's much deeper. The synchrony has to be there. Orgasms are achieved by your partner feeling they can trust you to sexually arouse them. Connect with your partner at an intimate level and the orgasm will come naturally. Women, for the most part, do not really place much concern on the size of the penis. Therefore, it is better to avoid placing emphasis on comparisons. Marriage is much more than that.

It is important to note that sex life changes as people age in a marriage. Surveys conducted indicate that as couples age in marriage, the average number of times they have sex a year decreases with time. The interesting fact is that it should not be interpreted as dissatisfaction. Most of the couples say that they are still satisfied and that they did not feel that the 'grass is greener on the other side'. This implies that sex life in marriage evolves for the better and couples should not try to be like they were in the past. Change is normal and should be expected as long the communication aspect of the marriage keeps getting better. Communication allows partners to discover what ignites that spark in their hearts and minds. It could be that it just needs going out on a romantic dinner or just as simple as taking a bubble bath together.

Sex also needs to have an element of unpredictability in a marriage. Romance and intimacy require breaking the habit of being too predictable. Falling into a comfort zone is often the case with couples but much more is needed if strengthening of the bond has to happen. It may help if partners to make a list of things they would like to venture into in the bedroom or elsewhere and place them in a jar. Every time they get an idea, they put it down and place it in the jar. Every week, they can dip their hands in the jar and do what the fantasy requires. This reignites the spark every time and the thought of not knowing what's next makes it even more worthwhile.

Chapter 3: How to Revive Intimacy

When one or both partners in a marriage or relationship are not happy, intimacy becomes a thing of the past. If one party isn't feeling loved, or doesn't feel as though the other finds them attractive anymore, instead of trying to improve themselves by dressing up or putting a bit more effort into their appearance, the opposite often occurs, making intimacy even less of an occurrence.

Other factors can contribute to the decrease of intimacy as well. These can include work, health, tiredness and children. To revive the intimacy in your relationship you need to put a bit of effort in, but it may not be as difficult as it seems.

Prioritize Your Relationship

With so many distractions and interferences in our day to day lives, it is easy to push aside the relationship. Often this is just because so many other things need to be done, and there doesn't always seem to be enough hours in the day. To revive the intimacy, one tip is to make your relationship a priority. Two or three times a week set aside a bit of time for you and your partner to be alone. It doesn't have to be a major event – it could just be going for a walk, having a coffee and a chat, or anything you might both enjoy. But you need to do it together with nobody else around. This will enable both partners to feel more connected to each other, and therefore increase the intimacy.

Flirt With Each Other

Remember back to when you first started dating, and how you used to flirt with each other. This shouldn't stop just because you are married – it should still be an important part of your relationship. Texts, emails or little notes to each other can be very stimulating on many levels. It will bring a smile to the recipient's face, and add a little anticipation to what may lie ahead at the end of the day. Flirting can also be successfully achieved by surprising your partner by dressing up more than usual. If they see you in your sweat pants on a daily basis, coming home to a wife dressed to the nines in a pair of heels will certainly get things going!

Create a Habit

A habit or a ritual that you do together can make each partner feel more connected to the other. For many couples, it is the simple ritual of kissing goodbye in the morning, and again when you see each other at the end of the day. But it can be any activity you wish, such as watching a regular television program together or saying I love you before you go to sleep at night. Whatever ritual you create, you need to follow it through every day.

Getting In the Mood

Sex drives can vary tremendously through different periods in our lives, and more often than not, one partner's drive will be higher than the other's. A lot of couples will just wait until they are both in the mood, but with the variance in the drives, this could go on for quite some time. So, you need to try and get yourself into the mood for sex regularly. This may mean exploring what it is that arouses you, or makes you feel sexy.

Date Nights

This is becoming more and more popular, and it's a great way to have some time alone together whilst doing something enjoyable. Think back to what you used to do before jobs, mortgages and kids came along. Go out to your favorite restaurant, or send the kids to the grandparents and have a candlelit dinner at home. Nothing provokes intimacy more than good food, soft music and candlelight. Or, if you are more of the adventurous couple, go out and do an activity you will both enjoy. Perhaps you could both go to dancing lessons once a week, or go see a movie. Just so long as you do something together once every week to keep those sparks going.

Make Them Feel Special

It's the little things in life that you can do for one another that can make your partner feel more special and loved. Think about something they really like, and surprise them with it without them having to ask for it. This could be cooking them their favorite dinner, serving breakfast in bed, or maybe getting that new book they wanted to read. If you are leaving the house before them, leave them a little note telling them to enjoy their day and that you love them. Letting your partner know you love them and doing little things for them will make them feel special and increase the intimacy between you.

Terms of Endearment

How many couples, when they first started dating, came up with pet names for each other? These terms of endearment are special and intimate, and there is no reason why they shouldn't continue throughout your marriage. It doesn't have to be some crazy little nickname like snuggle bunny; it could just be a name like dear, or darling. When you started out in your relationship, that nickname was brought about by how you felt about your partner. Continuing to use it reminds them that you still feel that way. It's also very important to tell your partner you love them regularly. We often lose sight of that, and being reminded that you are loved can be a great boost to any marriage.

Don't Let Yourself Go

This is just as important for women as it is for men. Yes, it's true that it can be difficult to maintain an ideal physical image, particularly as we age, or as life becomes busy. But, it is nice for both partners to see their significant other making a bit of effort to look good. You don't have to look like a superstar of course, but you shouldn't spend days on end in the same clothes with your hair in a mess either! More often than not, when you put a bit of effort into your appearance it can do wonders for your self-esteem, and that alone can make you more desirable to your partner.

Don't Take Arguments to Bed

The bedroom is the place in your house that should be reserved for showing affection and love to one another, so it shouldn't be tainted by ongoing disputes or arguments. Make a pact with your partner that you will always try to resolve any issues before you even enter the bedroom. Don't go to sleep angry, as you will still feel the same in the morning. Also, by carrying an argument into the bedroom, you will find you drift apart in the bed, and with no cuddling, caressing or pillow talk, this will create a divide between you and ruin the intimacy.

Increase Your Physical Contact

A little touch from your partner here or there throughout the day and evening can invoke a sense of intimacy. It could be a simple touch on the back in passing, or more involved such as a neck massage. The neck is quite a sensuous part of the body, and the massage works by relaxing the muscles and therefore relaxing the body. This relaxation technique can help get you in the mood for intimacy.

Chapter 4: Creating Emotional Intimacy with Your Man

If you want to create emotional intimacy, you need to lay the groundwork and actually see how he is *responding* to it. If you've been reading this book, you've likely figured out that creating this environment fertile to emotional intimacy is a lot of work.

But how do you know if he's responding the way you want? It can be difficult.

When you voice your emotions to your partner, how does he react?

If you are upset or angry or happy or nervous, you should put these feelings to direct words. Again, expecting him to read your mind is a one-way ticket to disaster.

However, when you voice your feelings... how does he react? Does he react with positive affirmations, or at least acknowledgment? Or does he seem disinterested? In healthy emotional relationships, partners at least acknowledge each other's feelings, even if they don't agree with them. If your man seems distant or completely uninterested in what you're feeling, that's a danger sign.

On the flip side, if you want to create an environment of emotional intimacy, you need to acknowledge when your man speaks to you about his emotions. Many men love it when their female partners act as an emotional sounding board. It makes them feel loved and appreciated.

Communicate directly with him. Again. Do not hint. If you want to spend more time with your man, do not attempt to do this by making him *jealous* by flirting with other men at the bar. This sends mixed signals and will absolutely not get you the response that you want.

If you express yourself in a clear and positive manner, you will get the results you want. Likewise, don't take his truthfulness as a personal attack. If you ask him how that dress looks on you and he doesn't like the dress... don't fly off the handle at him about it. You asked, and he responded. It doesn't mean he thinks you are unattractive. He simply didn't like the dress.

If you can engage in clear and constructive conversation and criticism of each other, it will actually deepen your intimacy because both of you know that your opinions are safe with each other.

Accept him and do not try to change him. Women are notorious for trying to mold their men into perfect relationship-material, and *this does not work*. The only person that you can change is yourself. Of course, there are some examples of this. If your man is a smoker and he decides that he wishes to quit, you can absolutely emotionally support him through being weaned off nicotine.

However, in this example, you are *helping* your man change in a way that he has decided on his own to do. If he doesn't want to quit smoking, demanding that he stop because *you* want him to is ineffective. Either accept that your man smokes cigarettes, or consider it a deal-breaker and move on.

This also goes with emotions. If you tell your man that you really, really like him and he changes the subject or looks uncomfortable or otherwise does not respond with the same amount of affection that you do... do not try to get him to "love you more." This has to happen at its own pace. If it isn't happening, it isn't.

Likewise, if you want to create that awesome environment of intimacy, you definitely need to reciprocate his own displays of affection! If he tells you he loves you or adores you or wants you, make sure to tell him back in kind if you feel the same way!

Be open about sex. Obviously, if you want to fuck his brains out you need to be open and engaged with sex. However, it's important to figure out how both you and he react to each other in this manner. Do you feel inhibited or shy when bringing something up to him that you desire sexually? Are you hoping that sex will actually translate into him spending more time with you or giving you the affection that you crave?

Sex should be about sex alone. It is not a weapon that should be used to hurt your man, and it's not an item that should be exchanged for other commodities like love. You also should feel free to talk to your partner about your sexual desires. Of course, different people have different sexual desires - some may feel that mild bondage is extremely kinky, while others already have a dungeon set up in their basement for play.

The idea is not that you and your man can't have limits on what you will or won't do during sex, but that you are okay with talking about sex and you don't feel as though you'll be judged for bringing up things that you desire. For instance, some people couldn't imagine a sex life without anal, while others find the entire concept disgusting. For a great sex life, you need to be compatible in this manner.

Chapter 5: Spice Things Up In the Sack

It can be easy to fall into the same-old-same-old when it comes to sex with your man, and that's not good for him or you. You can ensure to keep on blowing his mind by keeping things a little more interesting. If you're not sure where to start, we can help you out with that!

Get all dressed up. Nothing like a little bit of clothing fun to make things a bit different. Lingerie is probably the most traditional thing here, but you can always make it a bit more exciting with French maid costumes or the like. Don't forget that he can always get dressed up, too! Maybe he could dress up like a sexy air conditioner repairman. (Just a suggestion.)

Don't look away. The next time you have sex with your man, try keeping your eyes open the entire time. You may not even realize it, but you very likely have a tendency to close your eyes during sex and escape off into your own little world. If you keep your eyes focused on your partner during sex, you may very well be surprised at how intimate the moment can become.

(Hey, spicing it up isn't *just* about getting wilder than normal! Getting more emotionally intimate than normal can be extremely powerful!)

Get down with the Kama Sutra. There's a reason why this book has been around for centuries, and it's largely because it has a bunch of amazing sex moves in it. Some of the moves in the Kama Sutra are... astoundingly complex and probably shouldn't be attempted unless you are a gymnast, but there are some that are considerably more doable in nature.

For instance, consider trying **making a fire**, where you rub your husband's erect penis like you're trying to start a fire with a stick. You may also try **spiraling the stalk**, which is where you put one hand on top of another and twist them in opposite directions. **The thousand yonis** is a move where you put one hand on the top of his penis and stroke down, followed immediately by the other hand. Repeat with the first hand over and over. "Yoni" is the Sanskrit word for "vagina," and this move supposedly feels like he's entering a thousand different vaginas!

Again, these don't require an Olympic background in gymnastics to complete and are certainly an interesting twist on the same tired old handjob.

Don't feel as though you have to spend a lot of money to try something new. You may be a bit hesitant to drop a paycheck on a sex toy emporium, but you can definitely get kinky without having to spend a mint. For instance, common items around the house that can be used for a spanking scene involve spatulas, pans, spoons, or ping-pong paddles. You can try using a rolling pin to give massages. Heck, go into your laundry room while your dryer is set to tumble and take a tumble yourself on top of it!

Bring food into it! Food play is simple, sexy, and fun. Try covering your man in chocolate or whipped cream or pudding or anything you'd like to lick and then lick it off of him in lines. You can also feed chocolate-dipped fruit to each other. (The only thing to be careful of is sugary items around your vagina. If sugar gets into your vagina it becomes a prime breeding ground for yeast, which you definitely want to avoid.)

Try some light bondage. There are indeed people out there who are into their chains, but if those are just too intimidating for you, there are other, lighter ways to make it work. Consider using neckties or scarves to tie wrists or ankles together. If you're really nervous, you can just wrap them around your wrists and hold the ends of the ties in your hands. If you want to get into bondage a little more seriously but not spend a lot of money, consider investing in zip ties. They are virtually unbreakable and very inexpensive. (Just make sure to wrap a scarf or sock around body parts first so that the zip tie doesn't accidentally cut too much into the skin.)

Put on a show for your partner. Masturbating in front of your partner isn't just a way to turn him on, but it's also a great way to show him what you do when you're alone. After all, you definitely know what you like, right? Show your partner and you'll reap the benefits! It's also very educational for you as well to watch your man masturbate. And even if you've never thought of that being a sexy thing to watch, you may be surprised. You like to watch your man in pleasure when he's having sex with you, right? It's also fun to watch him in the throes of pleasure when he's going at it solo!

Consider toys. Again, they aren't necessary, but they *can* up your game to a whole other level. You don't need to go with giant rubber penises or massive vibrators, either. There are tons of much more discreet products to choose from if you're a bit hesitant. There is also a wide *array* of products for you to choose from, including things like Ben Wa balls or anal beads or cock rings. The options are literally endless so get on the internet and do some research. If you're not shy, you can go to your local sex shop and see what they have on display.

Share your fantasies with each other. As mentioned earlier in the book, if you feel hesitant to talk about your sexual fantasies with your partner, that's a bad sign. Additionally, just because you *talk* about your fantasies does not mean that you have to actually act them out. (And depending on the fantasy, fulfilling it may not be possible, anyway. Your man may have a thing for 20-armed tentacle monsters, but even if you were down with the same thing it would be rather hard to find a tentacle monster to play with.)

The simple act of sharing may turn you on and get you closer. Not to mention, simply talking about sex may be enough to make you hot.

Talk dirty to him. Most men love phone sex. Even if you're going to see each other later on tonight, there's no reason not to engage in a bit of afternoon delight with him on his lunch break. This will turn him on early in the day and keep you on his mind until he gets home at night. If you can't bring yourself to actually utter the words on the phone (or if you're in an area that is too public for dirty talk), send some sexy texts.

Consider sexy pictures. Many women aren't comfortable with sending nudes to their men, but men definitely love it when women do. So go find a room with favorable lighting and get your selfie on. Another great idea is to have your partner take pictures of you, or perhaps videotape having sex together. Men, in particular, are very visual creatures, so having lots of visual stimulation of you on hand is a sure way to get you into his mind. Also considering asking *him* to send *you* some sexy pictures. This isn't as common, but most men are very happy to oblige!

Don't get scripted. Sex is wonderful when it's spontaneous! Make sure that you sometimes jump him when he gets out of the shower or right when he walks in the room. Many people get in the trap of scheduling their sex like it's an errand, rather than a true expression of love and affection. Keep your man guessing, and make it clear that you're open for unexpected advances on his part as well. This will keep your sex life fresh and exciting.

Consider investing in a book collection. Books like this can help you keep things exciting and give you ideas for when you get stuck in a rut. But don't feel as though you have to be consigned solely to advise books! Getting great sexual fantasy literature will give you great ideas as well.

Watch porn together. While many women don't exactly like visual pornography all that much, it's a rare man who does not. Even if you're not that into porn yourself, consider watching it with your man. He will likely find it an unbelievable turn on, and it may be a source of new ideas, just like your book collection is.

Don't get focused on the end goal. Even if you have the most amazing sex life in the world, both partners are not going to orgasm all the time. You may be under stress or your body just isn't feeling it that day for whatever reason. This can also happen with him - he's not a sex machine either. Don't be goal-oriented when it comes to sex; be experience-oriented. You can have an encounter where you, your man, or both you and your man do not orgasm and that doesn't make the sex bad.

Laugh. Sex is funny. You'll make funny noises and occasionally you'll be in the middle of a complicated move when he rolls over onto his car keys, gets poked in the ass, and loses his erection. It happens. Also, make sure to engage in playful acts that may not be directly sex-related. For instance, try buying body paint or playing strip Twister or something like that. This will keep your sex lives more fun, and create that environment of intimacy where both of you will be more inclined to trust and engage with the other.

Chapter 6: Communication Practices

The absolute greatest sex – by far – happens between two people who care about each other's pleasure equally and unselfishly.

If you want to have great sex, throw out your ego, throw out any self-absorption you have in your sex life, and throw out any sexual selfishness.

Communication must begin from a place of mutual caring for each other's pleasure and satisfaction, from a place of vulnerability, and most importantly, from a place of trust. Only from there can one's sex life reach astronomical heights.

Communication is harped on constantly in sex articles on the internet. But they rarely go farther than, "You should communicate with your partner about what you like and don't like, and be attentive to your partner's needs." While this is true, it goes much deeper than that.

Having sex is one of the most vulnerable acts you can do with another person. All of your insecurities, all of your anxieties, all of your stress about your performance, your body image, your past experiences – they can all converge in the bedroom.

When communicating with your partner, try your best to practice empathy. Try your best to put yourself in their shoes and see things from their perspective. And if they aren't doing this for you, let them know that you would like them to.

It's also important to set up boundaries in the bedroom, especially when you get deeper into sexual fantasies and the kinkier stuff. It takes a long time to build trust in one another, so that trust should be held sacred.

Here's a comment from a Redditor that applies to this topic:

"Trust in the bedroom builds up over time and can be taken away in a second. Define what trust means in and out of the bedroom."

And another Redditor talking about discussing sex with your partner:

"Also, I think that some people may experience awkwardness talking about sex. It's not always easy to discuss casually, we're so afraid of hurting people's feelings or feeling judged."

I think both of these comments hold true.

You may want to tell your partner that you don't like something they've been doing in bed for months, but you haven't had the heart to hurt their feelings. You have decided to keep it inside, but it's becoming a bigger and bigger issue for you. It's hard to bring these things up with someone you care about, and even more difficult to say it in a way that doesn't hurt their feelings.

You may also want to try something new, but this "something" has been deemed "weirder" by societal standards or is not as common, making you feel like you can't talk about it. But it has been eating away at your thoughts and your fantasies. You want to discuss trying it with your partner. You just don't know-how. You don't want them to judge you.

I have laid out exact scripts and worksheets you can use to work through this communication with your partner. I'm framing them in a letter format because going through dialogue wouldn't provide as good of an example.

You can use these as samples or follow them exactly. Either way, they should help ease the process. I have also included some helpful considerations to keep in mind when discussing these issues.

Script #1 – Discussing Something You Want to Try

There's something I've been meaning to talk to you about, but I've been holding off on it because it makes me feel a little uncomfortable. I'm more comfortable with you than I have been with anyone else, so I'm going to push through and say it anyway.

It's about something I've been wanting to try in the bedroom. It's not exactly something that our friends have done, and it makes me feel weird just thinking about it. But it has been eating away at my thoughts and I can't keep it in any longer. And most importantly, I want to try it with you, because I trust you so much and my feelings for you are so strong.

I want to try being handcuffed *(note: or whatever you want to try)*. I know you're not into being dominant, but I would love for you have total control over me in the bedroom, at least once, just to see how it is. If you do this for me, I would love to do something for you as well. It'll be like a trade!

Either way, if you are absolutely not comfortable with it, that is totally fine. I don't want you to feel pressured into it, and I wouldn't want to feel that way myself. But I do think it would be something fun to try. If we end up hating it, we can stop immediately. And if we end up loving it, awesome!

Let me know what you think.

Keep in mind-

- Your partner may be uncomfortable with what you want to try, so communicate that you understand this.
- Let them know this isn't something you want to do with just anyone, but that you want to share it with them and them alone (I get that this won't be totally true all the time, but it makes it more special).
- Try to see your request from your partner's perspective, and be empathetic to how they may feel about it.
- Don't pressure them. The more you pressure them, the easier it will be for them to deny your request and more conflict will arise. Give

them a way out by saying if they're too uncomfortable, it's okay and it won't change the relationship.

- If your partner is making this type of request to you, imagine that you had a burning desire to try something. Step into your partner's shoes. Think about how you would want your partner to react. Then react accordingly.

Script #2 – Telling Your Partner That You Don't Like Something They Do in Bed

Our sex life is absolutely amazing. You're a freak in bed and you turn me on so much. I get horny just thinking about you as I go about my day.

I love everything you do in bed, especially when you pull my hips into you whenever we have sex *(or whatever you genuinely love about what they do)*. But there's just one thing that I know you like to do, and it's really hot, but it actually kind of hurts me *(or the reason why you don't like it)*.

I wish it didn't, but I can't control it. And I don't want you to feel bad thinking that it's your fault or anything. It's something neither of us can control.

When we're in that position where you're on top of me, and you roll your hips side to side, it feels really good for the most part, except it hurts my lower back quite a lot. I think it's from an old injury I got in high school, but it's pretty painful.

I don't mean to make you feel bad, because if it wasn't for my back, I would love it 100%. You look so hot when you're rolling your hips like that. But it hurts enough to where it totally distracts me from your sexiness.

I know I can't be a complete saint, so if there is anything I'm doing that you don't like, feel free to tell me. I'd rather both of us openly communicate like this and get these things out of the way, than stay silent doing things in the bedroom that actually hinder our sex life.

Keep in mind-

- Your partner may love doing the thing you don't like, and may think that you love it as well. If this is the case, some of their sexual ego and self-esteem may be tied to this act. So let them know the reason(s) why you don't like it, as gently as you can.

- Compliment them on the things you like first. Make them genuine comments. There's no use in communication if you are going to lie and fabricate things. Be honest, but be tactful in your honesty.

- Extend the lines of communication by being open to finding out something they don't like which you do in bed. This makes it more of an open forum, rather than one person being targeted.

Script #3 – Discussing a Fantasy You Have

This is something I have never shared with anyone. I only think about this when I am by myself, and I've kept it a secret for years.

But I want to share it with you because I trust you not to judge me, even if you don't want to try it.

I have this sexual fantasy. It feels weird for me to actually explain it out loud, so please, don't make fun of me. It's a fantasy where you knock on the front door and pretend like you're delivering a package *(insert whatever fantasy you have)*. We don't know each other, but when we see each other, we're immediately attracted to one another.

You say it's hot outside, so I invite you in for a drink. But next thing I know, you grab my face, pull it into yours, we start kissing, and eventually stumble into the bedroom and have sex.

I know it sounds a little funny, and it's not like I would want something like that to happen in real life. But I feel so comfortable with you, so pretending like we didn't know each other would be really hot for me.

How do you feel about it?

I also want you to feel comfortable telling me any fantasies you have that you would like to act out. We might as well get them all out in the open and see which ones we want to try. I think it could be really fun. What do you say?

Keep in mind-

- Fantasies can be uncomfortable to discuss, whether they are your own or your partner's. However, they are also completely natural. Pretty much everyone has them. So try to create an environment of understanding in which to let them out.
- Invite your partner to share their fantasies as well.

Script #4 – Talking About Your Insecurities and Anxieties

I wish this didn't bother me, but I can't help it. I feel really insecure about it and it makes me extremely anxious. It's got to do with something we do in the bedroom.

Up until now, I haven't said anything. I know I should have said something in the beginning, and that's my mistake, but I didn't want you to feel like I was taking something away from you. I also know that it's my insecurity and I have to deal with it myself, but it's gotten to a point where I can't do it anymore – at least not for a while until I work through it.

Using the dildo on you makes me very uncomfortable. It's bigger than me, and I'm scared you might like it more than me. I know this is crazy, because that thing is a piece of rubber. But I can't help it. Every time we use it, it makes me feel so uncomfortable.

I know that it's something you enjoy, and to think that a toy could replace me is nuts. But it's an insecurity I have been dealing with my whole life. I hope you can understand that.

I am totally open to other toys, so if there is something else you want to try in the meantime, I'm all ears. I just can't use that one anymore. I'll get through it eventually, but for now, it's causing me too much stress.

Thanks for being so understanding. If you have something you would like to talk about, I promise I won't judge you either and I'll do my best to help you through it.

Keep in mind-

- Insecurities run deep. They can cause people intense amounts of stress and anxiety, especially when it comes to sex.
- In the present, insecurities are largely uncontrollable. It takes time to work through these things. So if your partner suddenly brings up something they would like to stop doing in bed, don't take it personally. This may be something they have been dealing with for years, and it may have been hard to talk to you about it.
- Also, don't be afraid to express your insecurities. Often, one of the best ways to get through them is simply to let them out.

> Tell them to someone you trust and who cares about you. They may be able to provide a different perspective to help you out.

- Once again, maintain an open forum. When expressing an insecurity, your partner may be harboring their own. Give them an opportunity to express theirs as well so you can work through each other's together.

Establishing Boundaries

Knowing each other's boundaries is an essential part of communication. This is where you really get to know your partner's likes, dislikes, and subtle sexual tendencies. These play out in the bedroom constantly, so it's important that you're attentive to them.

I understand this is harder to do with casual relationships and one-night stands. Sometimes the nature of the relationship dictates that this stuff isn't communicated.

What you can do is a simplified version of what I'm about to show you. You would do everything verbally, and usually right after or right before having sex. Then, if you end up having sex again, you will understand much more about your partner's desires, your partner will understand much more about your own, and it will materialize itself into better sex.

I got this idea from a commenter on Reddit. The commenter noted that when she first got together with her partner of 10 years, she wrote out a list of things for them to discuss their sex life. Each item was rated on a scale of 1-10. Afterward, they could swap papers, compare answers, and have a much more open and structured discussion about their sex life.

They also came up with a sexual bucket list, which can give partners goals to strive for and make trying new things more fun. I think both of these ideas are brilliant.

Using these two ideas, you can gain a number of things:

- Knowledge of what your partner likes and dislikes.
- What boundaries you should stick to.
- A platform for open communication.
- Goals to work towards together.
- A way to communicate without actually having to say anything, which can make it easier to get started.

I've come up with two sample lists, one including topics for discussion where you would provide a rating for each, and another with possible goals for a sexual bucket list.

I suggest using these as a guide, creating your own, and trying them out. You never know how much it could deepen your connection and improve your communication skills.

Topics for discussion (the first four came from the Redditor)-

1. What level of trust do you have for your partner in the bedroom?
2. How kinky are you?
3. How kinky do you think your partner is?
4. How kinky are you willing to go for your partner?
5. How comfortable are you talking openly about sex?
6. How much do you enjoy giving oral sex?
7. How much do you enjoy receiving oral sex?
8. How much foreplay do you like, 1 being "not very much" and 10 being "a lot"?

9. How willing are you to try anal sex?

10. How willing are you to try having sex in public?

11. How willing are you to try experimenting with sex toys?

12. How comfortable do you feel with being vocal in the bedroom?

13. How comfortable do you feel being constrained by your partner?

14. How comfortable do you feel being blindfolded?

15. How comfortable do you feel watching porn with your partner?

16. How comfortable are you discussing sexual fantasies?

17. How comfortable are you acting out sexual fantasies?

18. How much do you enjoy being more dominant?

19. How much do you enjoy being more submissive?

20. How much do you struggle with sexual anxiety and insecurity?

When you print it out, write a number from 1 to 10 next to each question. Each partner should fill out their own answer sheet.

Afterward, switch papers and read over your partner's answers. Then discuss each answer. Along the way, you will figure out where your partner's boundaries lie and where to go from there.

Example Sexual Bucket List-

- Have sex on the beach
- Perform oral sex while driving
- Have sex in the backseat of a car
- Have sex on the kitchen floor
- Use a toy on each other at the same time
- Take a trip to the sex shop together
- Watch porn together
- Play a sexual card game
- Have sex four times in one day (or as many as you desire)
- Have sex in the shower

- Perform/receive oral sex in the shower
- Have sex with the curtains open
- Have sex while watching a movie
- Read an erotic book together
- Try constraining each other
- Fulfill one fantasy of each partner
- Research tantric sex together
- Try five new positions every month
- Have anal sex
- Surprise one another with a sexual gift
- Add multitasking into the bedroom
- Have a threesome
- Try switching dominant and submissive roles
- Have sex in every room of the house
- Have sex every day for a month straight
- Have morning sex every day before work for a month straight
- Have sex while cooking dinner
- Have sex while eating dinner
- Make a porno together

Each partner would create their own, switch with their partner, then collaborate with each other on what they want to pursue.

Applying the Communication Principles

The biggest part of communication is practicing empathy. You have to try your best to see where your partner is coming from, and they should do the same for you.

The next big thing is being open and honest with your partner. It's okay if you feel uncomfortable. These things are inherently uncomfortable, **but that's why it is so important to talk about them.**

Bottling up these thoughts and feelings doesn't do you any good.

Expressing them does you a world of good and will bring you and your partner closer together. You may also experience some of the craziest sex of your life. And all you had to do was tell your partner you wanted to try something new.

Communicate with empathy, communicate honestly and openly, establish boundaries, and write out your desires.

Ba da bing, ba da boom. Great sex awaits.

Chapter 7: Forgetting About Past Ghosts

We all sometimes think about the past for different reasons; it is completely normal to think about it, and sometimes, it is even inevitable. However, there is a point where we need to stop thinking about it so much or avoid doing it all together. That is when it keeps bringing us bad memories that are preventing us from enjoying our present and preventing us from moving on.

When positive things come to our mind, thinking about past experiences doesn't bring any negative effects; but when these thoughts tend to come with any signs of sadness, anger or distress, it might be better to leave them buried in time. It is important to remember that the unpleasant experiences we had are now behind us and even if they hurt at the time, we cannot let them hurt us forever. The truth is that bad things happen to everyone. Some of these things are worse than others, and some are harder to forget; but it is important to move on without letting those experiences drag us down. If we constantly let our memories haunt us, then we are the ones sabotaging ourselves. There is no doubt that sometimes our past can affect our present and our future, and that is why we need to cut those chains, and you are the only one that can do that. Nobody else but ourselves can control our minds and thoughts so slowly, but surely we need to train ourselves to block those things that come with repercussions.

There are many things from the past that can affect us. These are the most common ones: past experiences, past comments, or people. All of these things have the potential to affect us significantly and in some cases, it is hard to just let these things go. Sometimes it is difficult, and you might think it is impossible to let whatever that is affecting you go, but we need to do it, sometimes all together or sometimes step by step. And the first step is to understand how much your life can improve if you don't focus on these pasts ghosts. If we let these things bother us constantly, they can affect our self-esteem, the ability to trust, our relationships with others, our plans, and many other things. You might not think it is that important or that deep, but whatever that is negative can affect you somehow. So you need to find a way to move away from that in order to have good relationships with others and with yourself.

We are going to be focusing on the times that past ghosts affect our emotional, physical and sexual life. If your relationship is being affected by something from the past, there are two possibilities. (A) What is affecting you is related to an experience you went through while in the relationship. Something that your significant other did or said that ended up hurting you and caused issues in the relationship. (B) Something that happened in the past that is not related to your partner but still manages to affect your relationship. Whether your case is A or B, you need to know that you are not the only person that has ever been affected by any of these; luckily, it is never too late to try to move forward.

Being affected by something that happened during our marriage

Marriages are complex; they are full of ups and downs. Therefore, there is going to be more than one occasion that has certain experiences that hurt to remember. We need to consider something, however. If you are still with someone, it is because you decided to be with them regardless of anything else that might have happened between the two of you. If you decided to forgive your spouse because of something they said/did, then you need to try to get over that dark experience. Basically, you need to forgive and forget. It is not enough with you doing the first one, you need to try and do the two of them. We understand that forgetting something, especially something painful is not that simple, and the truth is we might not be able to forget about it completely because it might still run through our head from time to time. However, we need to stop giving it importance. Don't spend any time thinking about it. Any time that this bad memory pops up, you need to eradicate it, and think about something good instead. Even if it's still in your mind, try not to speak about it. Constantly bringing up the past can be equally damaging to a relationship. When you are trying to construct something positive, you don't need a constant reminder of the negative things. This is bad for both parties; the other person will constantly feel accused and they will eventually feel like every attempt is in vain, and that no matter how hard they try to amend things, they will always be attacked because of the past. Also, the person who is bringing it up will never be able to get healed and will start exhibiting toxic behaviors in the relationship, even though in their head, they think they are the victims. Whether what happened between you and your partner was something big or small, pointing fingers forever, especially after coming to an agreement to try to fix things, is very unhealthy. If the actions that hurt you are small issues, then think that it is not worth to bring your relationship down for something that is meaningless. If your relationship was affected by something more serious, the fact that both of you decided to overcome it and keep trying, speaks a lot. If you didn't let adversity break you down, do not let past memories do so.

Being affected by something that happened outside or before our marriage

It is common to be haunted by painful memories that happened before/outside our marriage, or things that don't have anything to do with your spouse, but still somehow affect our relationship. Things that cause us great pain, no matter how deep into the past they are, can still manage to affect different aspects of our lives; but we need to let those things go for our own good and for the good of people around us. We deserve to be happy and not let anybody or anything that is no longer relevant still take a toll on our well-being. If you keep bringing these things up and bringing insecurities into your life, this is going to affect your relationship with others as well, including your relationship with your spouse. You can count on your spouse to help you, and that is absolutely fine. Be honest with your spouse. Let them know about those things that affect you, and ask them to help you leave those issues behind. Couples are there to support each other, and facing things together is the best way to overcome problems. What is not okay, however, is to blame our spouse for things they are not guilty of. As an example, let's say that in the past you were with a partner that was unfaithful to you and now you think that your current partner will also be unfaithful even if they have done nothing to make you believe this. You can't just assume that everybody's the same. Just because someone said or did something, doesn't mean someone else is going to do it as well. You cannot put everybody into the same category. Your spouse is not guilty or responsible for the things that you might have experienced in the past, so why hold grudges against them? Past events sometimes bring insecurities, and it is understandable; but attacking people because of your insecurities is not alright. Do not forget that sometimes, instead of judging others, we need to judge ourselves. We have all the right to be happy, so don't be the one who is actually getting on the way.

The ways those past ghosts can affect your relationship

- You hold anger towards your significant other for something that happened between the two of you in the past.

- You cannot stop thinking about the negative experiences from the past.

- Bad thoughts related to past experiences are preventing you from expressing yourself the way you would like to sexually/romantically.

- You feel that you cannot forgive your significant other for something they did/said.

- You can't trust people, including your significant other, for something someone else did/said.

- You constantly victimize yourself.

- You are stuck to the past.

- You don't believe people can change.

If you identify yourself with one of the problems mentioned above, then it's most than likely that your relationship is currently being affected by past grudges. We have previously spoken about the reasons why you might be feeling this way, and the importance of not letting things get in the way, as well as how to stop them from doing so. However, we understand that sometimes, things are not that easy to see; but even if you only suspect that your relationship is being affected, it is good to put the things you learned into practice. You don't have to wait until things aggravate more. In fact, the sooner you tackle a problem, the better.

The moment something gets in the way of you being able to enjoy your emotional, physical, and sex life with plenitude, it is the moment you need to consider this as a problem. It is not fair for us or for our spouse to prevent ourselves from living the kind of relationship we would like to have, just because we cannot move on.

Having a relationship is easy, but in order to have a healthy and strong relationship, the people involved have to work hard and be able to enjoy every aspect of the relationship.

The ghost of previous relationships and experiences

We all have a past and it is completely normal to have had a romantic and a sexual life before being with the person you're currently with. We can't deny what had happened, but that does not mean we have to constantly bring it up. Many relationships suffer from a very unpleasant problem of having to constantly hear about exes, deal with them or even worse, being compared to them.
It is not okay to compare people; it is disrespectful and it can cause harm, although some people don't seem to understand that. They think that doing so is completely innocent, but the truth is that even if your partner doesn't say anything to you, having to hear explicit details about your romantic or sexual life with someone else is never easy and it can be very off-putting. Even if your partner is a laid-back type of person who is not jealous and whom you feel that you can talk to about

anything, they still have feelings. You need to think before you speak. How would you feel if the situation was the other way around? At the end of the day, we can't read minds, and if you are constantly speaking about a person you were with before, that might set off some red alerts in your partner and bring some insecurities since they might feel you still think too much about somebody else, or still focusing on the past.

There are two scenarios when it comes to exes, you might still talk to them or you might not. If your ex is no longer part of your life, then let it go. Focus on the new chapter of your life, and focus on the special person that is now with you. On the other hand, if your ex is still part of your life, for whatever reason, maybe for personal choice or because of an obligation, then you need to draw a line. Your ex is not the person you are with; they are not your partner anymore. They are not the main priority in your life and you don't have to base your life decisions around them or let them interfere with your personal life. Even if your ex is a good friend of yours and someone you care for, they sometimes can overstep, so for the good of your new relationship, you must not let your ex interfere even if you think they are doing it in a good way. You and only you have got to decide what to do with your life, and letting exes get in the way might potentially damage your relationship. You are not obligated to cut contact with your previous partners. However, you must understand that the treatment between an ex and your spouse can't be the same. You must be patient and considerate with your significant other and understand why they might feel uncomfortable about your ex.

As we previously mentioned, sometimes people tend to compare their spouses with an ex or a previous partner and this can be very distasteful. We would recommend that you refrain from comparing, especially, if the comparison has to do with anything physical or sexual. Some people might think it is okay to compare especially if what they have to say favors their spouse; however, your point might come across better if you don't bring other people to the equation. There are other better ways to compliment someone. Try to do it in a way that will make your partner feel like they're the only person that you think about in that manner. Also, do not expect your partner to act the same way or do the same things that any of your previous romantic/sexual partners did. They are their own person and should not be held to previous expectations.

Be careful with expectations

Sometimes people have an idea of what being in a relationship is supposed to be like or how sex is supposed to be. Often, this idea is based on past experiences; things we have heard from others and even certain things such as the sexual content made available through the media. However, every relationship is different, and every person has their own interests and way of doing things. Your marriage is a unique experience in all of its branches and that includes sexual matters. Not everything that you hear from others would necessarily apply to you; have it in mind that if you hear it from someone else, that is from their own perspective and their criteria, which might be totally different from yours. Also, not everything you see from certain sexual content is realistic or accurate. So enjoy what you have, and if your sex life needs improvements, do it based on the needs and desires of the two of you. Have it in mind that the sexual content you see has a purpose, which is the purpose of entertaining. The people you see through that screen are after all doing a job; they have something to sell. They are not going to show you the not so glamorous parts of sex. Sexual content often does not equal what it is like to have sex in real life. If you are not comparing yourself to the people you see performing these acts, why comparing or expecting your partner to be like that, or to do what they do? Whether you watch this kind of content or not is completely up to you; many people do, some others don't. Nevertheless, if you are a viewer, it is okay to inspire yourself from certain things, but do not expect your sexual act to be exactly as you see it in a movie. Don't forget what reality is like. It is actually more common than it seems to hear people saying that addiction to sexual content has taken a toll, not only on their sex lives, but on their general well-being. Do not let other things interfere with your getting pleasure through actual contact, and between you and your loved ones.

The moment you make the relationship all about the two of you only, the moment that relationship will start blossoming.

Chapter 8: Loving Words Heal Relationships

The most dominant two phrases that heal a harmed relationship are additionally the two phrases that are hardest to state... "I'm Sorry" and "I was wrong"...This is basic in healing relationships for couples.

The motivation behind why these phrases are hardest to state is because we would prefer not to admit that we have caused whatever broke or harmed a relationship. More often than not, we say that it was the other person's deficiency. Also, we hang tight for that person to be the first to apologize. In any case, the apology never comes because the other person is likewise hanging tight for it.

What's more, we realize that relationships inside the family and outside of it sometimes end in light of the absence of this apology. We know many separations happen just because either never made a move to apologize.

For what reason is it so difficult to admit that we weren't right and to apologize? It is straightforward... that is human instinct, a shortcoming which puts us over the others. What we need is to defeat this commitment to self. This requires personal development, compassion, and thinking about the other. What's more, a necessary apology will reestablish that broken relationship.

It doesn't make a difference who fouled up when a relationship is broken. Significantly, we venture out. Remember that the other person feels a similar way. We should state something that can prompt healing, for example, "I'm sorry that we are having this issue. Would we be able to discuss making things right once more?"

Making a stride like this quite often prompts healing a broken relationship. Furthermore, more often than not, the conversation results in the two gatherings saying 'sorry,' and this typically leads in a more grounded relationship.

Any healing in a relationship for couples requires some forgiveness. This should originate from the heart before it is said in words.

One must be cautious about is that as it may, in communicating forgiveness. To state "I forgive you" amidst a battle may be misjudged as "You weren't right," and would compound the situation. We should say "I forgive you" just when the other person requests forgiveness. At that point, these become the ideal words. Mercy can heal the relationship as well as the bodies and the brains of the two persons.

Keep in mind, in healing relationships for couples, we as of now have the words. We need to state them.

Have an incredible relationship by utilizing words that heal

FALLING IN LOVE - THROUGH YOUR OWN LOVE WORDS

Regardless of whether you have begun to look all starry eyed at years prior, or hoping to become hopelessly enamored now, I can share with you some extremely sentimental approaches to share your emotions. Purchasing a love card, or a romantic ballad is excellent, in any case, words mean more when you get them directly from your own heart. You need to realize how to state what you might want to express. From that point forward, applying some inventiveness will make you incline that your beginning to look all starry eyed at just because.

- Address it with the right "pet name."
- Use detail, and don't be hesitant to get "mushy."

- Express yourself enthusiastically with love quotes
- Be inventive and unique include something new.

When writing to the love of your life, it is great to start it off with a pet name. Perhaps you have something that nobody else hears? This would be the ideal time to use it. This love letter will be among you and the one you love, so make it individual. A few people like to use (infant, sweetie, hun, and so on). I state if you have something nobody thinks about because it might be excessively humiliating this is the time to use it.

When writing a sentimental love letter, it is tied in with being mushy. Express yourself now with all the soft stuff that you typically don't state. Try not to keep down, after this is the thing that a love letter is about. Get energetic with your words, and let that individual recognize what your heart feels for them.

Presently, someplace in the middle of the letter, use their real name. You would prefer not to overdo it by a considerable amount of pet names, yet one to start, and real name in the middle ought to be great. Make sure to use love quotes all through this gem. Genuine romance does not come around over and over again. You need to make sure you treat it well and care for it while you have it. You're telling them you love them, with imaginative detail.

Include something new. Something you have not raised in quite a while, or at no other time. Demonstrate to them that something new emerges to you. State what your heart needed to shout, the day you realized you were in love. Connections can be precarious, yet if you enable yourself to recollect how much you are in love, you will do fine.

How to Express Love Words

Communicating with a person that you genuinely like them calls for the use of love words. Love is the single component that makes a society what it is. Without love, there is no life, and this is the motivation behind why words of love are significant. There are numerous things that best display love words, and when the name is referenced, many recognize what it implies. People use multiple ways and incorporate the words and, they can do it orally, or they can write it down. The vast majority when they were growing up, they used to write love letters to one another. Today, people keep on composing love letters. This is an instrument used to display love words. It is a rare occurrence natural to impart these words, and it calls for certified fondness. There is something men do that best express the words. Initially, understand that words are simply words if there is no activity to coordinate. This is likely the best thing about love. Love is best shown in any case when words are included. It affirms what there as of now is.

In this manner, if you wish to use the words, it is vital that you reexamine yourself and see if you love the person. Sentimental love between a man and a lady is the thing that I have portrayed above and a portion of the words that you will discover incorporate the accompanying. Dear sweetheart, nectar, my love, my dearest, and the list goes on. Love is dynamic, and people are inventive. New ages keep on concocting love words like baby, boo, and numerous others. When it comes to utilizing these words, it is vital that you ensure that the person you are communicating to gets it. When there is viable correspondence, you can likewise anticipate just useful things in your relationship. There are such vast numbers of love words that you can use and different societies, and even religions may decide the words. Different dialects will have their one of a kind arrangement of words. While you wish to express your love to somebody, it doesn't need to be sexual love. You can have respect for your children, guardians, sisters, etc. It is additionally extremely vital to express appreciation to such people, and many do it consistently.

Coming up are next to a portion of the words that people use to demonstrate their children love pumpkin, bear, love bear, daylight, baby, and the list goes on. You can think of your one of a kind words which can be a nickname at the same time, is equipped with love. It is important to be active in showing love to other people. In society, some people frequently feel dismissed. Such people might not have dear companions or family. Life is desolate when you have nobody to impart to and you ought to endeavor to make love any place and whenever conceivable. If you're the sort of person who isn't active in showing love, begin doing as such, and you don't need to write a love letter. It is the thing that you state and how you state it. Love can include numerous viewpoints and figure out how to radiate through your cooperative attitude.

Using Words of Love to Inspire the Relationship - 3 Tips for Men to Learn

Cherishing Love Inspires the Heart to Create Words that Gives Love its Life.

Relationships are a back and forth movement on the life of all of us as we clear our path through the riddles of life and of love. To live in the steady "fight," as some are inclined to call it, is to live in the bogus acknowledgment that in one way or another there are always victors and failures as we cross the minefield of love.

I come at it from an altogether different point of view as I take a gander at the words, we as a whole appear to use to get us to where we even have a relationship. Men, generally, need such a considerable amount of assistance in this field and typically wallow because of poor role models, societal impacts, peer pressure and only by and large sluggishness in needing to be something more with their words to their partner.

There is always a way out, yet numerous men neglect to search for the way in any case when it comes to talking love to their partner.

So, what are a few ways to make words mean things again with your partner? A couple of tips can always prove to be useful, right men?

Tip 1: Women need to hear your heart. Most likely one of the hardest things for men to do as a result of the reality they were never educated how to do as such.

Begin little here, folks — an all-around set note left before work can be an incredible begin. The significant thing to do here is to claim your powerlessness to share your heart NOW yet disclose to her that you are learning.

Tip 2: Not each cherishing word should lead to sex! What a stun man. Because you state something decent doesn't imply that the spoken words are S-E-X! Get over yourself. In some cases, the most sentimental things we do will never lead to sex, nor should they.

Tip 3: Love to love. Reevaluate your relationship as a way to love simply cherishing your partner. If you center around the quintessence of your identity as a team, the relationship will rule your faculties.

Keep in mind, men. You are more than what you at any point, though you were with your words. Presently, live that way.

At last, Love is All There is So Let Your Words be Your Beginning.

Chapter 9: What Women Want; What Men Want

Since men and women are wired differently, how they approach sex also differs. There are a number of things that both of them want, but they may not explicitly express the desire for such things, for one reason or the other. Partners should always remember to communicate and to always think of their partners' feelings.

Things Women Want:

- **Threesomes**

One of the surprising things that women want is threesomes. Usually, it is men who are supposed to be keen on having a threesome. However, many women have been known to have had fantasies about having a threesome with another female.

It is important to point out that even though some people may have such fantasies, not every one of them would find the fantasies as pleasurable if the couple decided to play out some of these fantasies out in real life.

Couples should also note that threesomes may complicate the relationship. They can lead to feelings of jealousy and insecurity from either of them. It is advisable to seek someone who is not close to any of you if you choose to walk down that path.

- **Role-Playing**

Women crave adventure, especially where romance and sex are concerned. Women are therefore more imaginative. Roleplay is one of the ways couples can spice up their sex lives, by using their imagination to maximize the sexual experience between them.

Role play is one of the best ways to break a sex life that has become routine. It adds a fresh approach to sex and creates a sense of excitement that both couples have not felt for some time.

You can add costumes to make the roles more authentic. Some women may want to be dominated, while others want to experience the feeling of being in control. However, if you chose to do it, both parties must always feel comfortable with the roles they play, otherwise it will not work.

- **Sex Toys**

Couples are encouraged to use sex toys, particularly when the woman cannot get orgasms when she is with her partner. There are sex toys that are specifically designed for couples.

- **Rough sex**

Some studies have shown that 57% of women love it a little bit rough in the bedroom. Most women who would love rough sex, like to play a submissive role. The intensity of it may vary, depending on the woman.

Some women like a little bit of roughness like grabbing her from the waist pulling her tightly towards you. Others may want an even more intense experience that may qualify as S&M. it is therefore advisable that couples talk about what makes either of them uncomfortable, before trying out new things in the bedroom.

Some commentators and writers have pointed out that some women may be reluctant to rough sex, because it may contradict feminism and women empowerment. Despite the fact that they fantasize about it, they feel it may undermine their position as an equal in a relationship.

However, nothing can be further from the truth. Rough sex, in this case, is more like role-playing. Taking a submissive position in the bedroom should not mean that you are less than your partner. In any case, many powerful men have for centuries sought out dominiatrix in brothels, in order to gain pleasure from this submissive position they assume.

What Men Want:

There are a few things men fantasies about. As stated earlier, they are often simple and direct. Despite the fact that these things seem simple and physical, they can go a long way in helping you get to new levels of excitement.

- **Initiate Sex**

Men find it very flattering when a woman initiates sex. It is generally expected that men would initiate sex. For that reason, many men secretly wish their wives would initiate sex. It excites men on several levels. One is compliments and reassures him that he is wanted and it makes him feel attractive.

It is surprising and exciting when the woman suddenly initiates sex. It does not have to be complicated. Simply making a move and expressing your desire either verbally or physically will be appreciated by most guys.

- **Try New Positions**

Just like initiating sex, it can be a real turn-on for him when she initiates new things in the bedroom. Some women have reservations about making this kind of move. They feel he may take it like she is cheating or that she is saying that he is not good enough in bed.

However, most mature men appreciate when the woman takes the initiative. Many men out there also find it somewhat flattering that she is keen on trying new positions with him in the bedroom.

- **Watching Her**

Men respond much more to visual stimuli than women do. Men are easily aroused by a woman dancing provocatively in front of him. She may also choose to touch herself in front of him, especially if this is something that also turns her on.

- **Compliments**

Men have an ego and this is also true when it comes to sex. Giving him compliments that say something about his skills is not only beneficial to him, but it can be helpful to the woman as well. There are many other things you can compliment him on, including his fit body, charm, or masculinity.

Chapter 10: Tips to Have More Intimacy in Every Situation

There are many ways to spice up your sex life, and as you learned there is a lot beyond the bedroom that can be done to enhance it as well. This chapter will explore some ideas of what you can do to make your sex life even better outside of the bedroom.

Do Fun Things Together

Doing fun things together allows you to increase your dopamine levels together as well. When you have fun together, it increases your closeness with one another and can enhance the joy you experience with each other. It adds a unique sense of intimacy to your relationship that cannot be added by sexual experiences.

Ideally, you want to have fun together in a way that gets your blood pumping and your adrenaline rushing. Going to an amusement park, ice skating, visiting an upbeat concert, or otherwise doing something fun and exciting can increase the happiness of your experience with one another. Having fun this way can add energy to your relationship that will carry into the bedroom and make sex even more enjoyable.

Kiss More Often

Many couples, especially those who have been together a while tend to kiss less often. Kissing is a highly romantic and passionate act and should be done regularly. Think about it, at the beginning of the relationship you likely kissed your partner a lot more frequently than you do now that you are more comfortable together. You want to start doing it more often.

When you are kissing more regularly, don't just increase the volume but also increase the passion in each kiss. There is no need to peck and go. Give the kiss a few moments and truly experience your partner with each kiss. You can include your hands and body as well, or even kiss in other intimate areas such as on the cheek, forehead or hand.

Recall What It Was Like to Meet

When you first met you likely spent a lot more time getting to know one another and a lot less time watching TV or doing other things to pass the time. You can spend some time asking each other questions about life, or even just reminisce on the days when you met each other. Getting to know each other all over again is a great way to rekindle the flame in a relationship.

The reality is that we don't all stay the same in life. Throughout your relationship, you and your partner will change several times over. Their preferences for certain things may change, and these are all great things to learn about each other all over again as you rekindle your love by communicating and asking questions.

Describe Your Sexual Fantasies

Many times, sex is just about the act and couples don't really speak a lot about sex outside of the bedroom. A great way to spark up a flame and add passion to your sex life is to talk about each other's fantasies and interests. This gives you an opportunity to get to know each other's sexual preferences more intimately which means that you can gain maximum enjoyment out of sex. It allows you to have a better idea of what your partner likes and what they don't like, and how you can make sexual experiences more enjoyable for them.

Keep the Mystery Alive

In relationships, it can be easy to get to know each other so intimately that there appears to be no mystery left in the relationship anymore. This can be counterproductive to the process of bringing romance back into your relationship. A lot of romance builds around mystery and the desire to know each other more intimately than you presently do. There are many ways that you can add mystery back into your relationship, even if you already know almost everything about each other. Using sentences that add mystery, clothes that spark intrigue and even simple texts that make the other partner wonder what you have planned for the evening can help add mystery back into the relationship.

When the mystery is present, the other person wonders about you. They start thinking about you and may even become obsessed with wanting to know what you have planned because they are curious. Curiosity is the key to creating mystery and getting your partner wondering about you and what you have to offer them that is unique from before.

Express Gratitude

A great way to help your partner feel cared for and show them how much they mean to you is to express your gratitude. Expressing gratitude takes very little time but can have a significant impact on the quality of your relationship. When people feel cared for and loved, they want to show more care and love to the one they feel for as well. This can increase the quality of your relationship, making you both feel more appreciated.

In relationships, the little things often get overlooked. People forget that the little things count and so they don't take the time to show appreciation and gratitude for them genuinely. Something as simple as "I really appreciate that you always support me in my decisions" or "I really appreciate that you make me breakfast each morning" can go a long way. Even though repeat activities can lead to things being expected, it is always good to show that you don't necessarily expect things to be done for you or in a certain way. Always show that you care about what your partner does in life and for you, as this will increase the quality of your time together and make you both feel more loved overall. When you feel more loved, the sparks will naturally fly in your relationship.

Don't Hold Grudges

Holding grudges can destroy relationships really quickly. When people hold grudges, they fail to let go of things that are no longer relevant, and it can lead to destruction in the relationship. You may feel that if you let go, it shows your partner that their mistake was acceptable, and for you, it may seem like you are allowing them to do it again. In reality, when you let it go, you are giving them permission to be human and make mistakes. It allows them the opportunity to see what they've done and make a change, knowing that you will appreciate the change wholeheartedly. It never pays to hold a grudge in your relationship.

Care About Self Care

How you care about yourself and how your partner cares about themselves is important when it comes to having a healthy relationship. A healthy relationship almost always leads to a healthy sex life, since your sex life is so closely linked to the health of your relationship. It is important that you both emphasize self-care and take the time to truly nurture your own needs before nurturing your partner's. Yes, before. You cannot pour out of an empty cup, and keeping your cup empty is not a favor to your partner. Instead, it is a drawback that will lead to your relationship falling apart.

Taking care of your own self can come in many ways. You should look towards developing a healthy relationship with yourself if you want to really get serious about self-care. Take yourself on dates, have alone time, and get to know yourself more. The added benefit of getting to know yourself more is that you learn things about yourself that you may not have known before. You can share these things with your spouse, thus expanding your realm of conversation topics and letting you continue to get to know each other, even long after the relationship has worn out its honeymoon phase.

There are many ways that you can spark romance back into your relationship outside of the bedroom. By having these types of activities present in your day-to-day life, you increase the amount of romance and intimacy that lies between you and your partner and it causes you both to become more eager about your sex life. A relationship that is rich outside of the bedroom is one that will be exciting inside of the bedroom.

When you are looking to cause sparks outside of the bedroom, you want to take your time and really get to know one another. Forget everything you've learned up until now and take the time to learn again. In many cases what you know now can be relevant but may no longer be the whole truth. People regularly change, and this can lead to there being a disconnection between what you are thinking and what your partner is wanting. By communicating, you can alleviate this disconnection and create a renewed sense of appreciation and romance between yourself and your partner.

Overall, the best thing you can do for your sex life is to nurture all areas of your relationship. The more successful your relationship is elsewhere, the more exciting your sex life will be. It creates a sense of deep knowing and trust that cannot be faked between two people. When this trust and love is present, the sex you experience will be unlike anything you have ever had before. Even relationships that have been alive for a long time can benefit from this type of rekindling.

Chapter 11: Restoring Intimacy in Your Marriage

No marriage is complete without intimacy. Intimacy is what brings spark and fire to a marriage. Intimacy leads to romance and romance is what entangles you two, turning two souls into one. Yes, this unification of your souls and bodies is what this next step is about and exactly what has been missing out in your dull marital life for a very long time. When you don't spend time together, the intimacy greatly reduces and without intimacy in a marriage, it is really hard to have a successful marriage. Therefore, to make your married life happy again, you need to bring back the 'intimacy' element in it. Here's how you can do that.

Focus on Your Appearance

To be intimate with your spouse, you need to entice them and for that, you need to look good. How long has it been since you focused on yourself? Take a good look at yourself in the mirror and you'll find out why your better half isn't attracted to you anymore. Yes, being into looks is something shallow, but good looks are what attract people. You become attracted to good-looking people and the same goes for your spouse too. So, if you want to seduce them, you need to dress up nicely, work on your hair and face and look your best.

Additionally, start exercising to shed off the few extra pounds you have gained. Most women don't want a pot-bellied man and most men would not want a woman with love handles. Furthermore, most people who are overweight have a low self-esteem and if you don't feel good about yourself, then you are unlikely to enjoy intimacy. Once you start making an effort towards looking better, your spouse will notice this and this is likely to re-ignite that spark and remind your spouse of the person they fell in love with.

Make a Happy Ritual

Experts say that most couples become so lost in their professional lives that they fail to make time for one another. They come home exhausted from work, rest a little, play with kids probably, eat something and go to bed to prepare themselves for another hectic day at work. This pretty much sums up their routine lives and when they eventually have time on the weekend, they just want to catch up on some more sleep. When they have no time for one another, the closeness between them slips away. However, in order to restore your marriage and bring back intimacy, it is critical to make time for one another and develop a happy ritual just for the two of you. A happy ritual refers to a ritual you and your spouse practice with each other at least once a day, so that you can find some time even if it is just for a few minutes to spend with your loved one.

For instance, a psychology teacher who experienced the same problem with his wife once created a happy ritual with his wife wherein the two danced on seeing one another. This gesture expressed their happiness on seeing one another and also helped them get a break from their monotonous routine. You could do something like this too or come up with a creative happy ritual wherein you both show your contentment for each other. You could sing songs to each other, or give each other big smiles, or say something beautiful to one another whenever you see each other after a long day at work.

Send Sexy Messages/Emails

You may have been together for quite some time; hence, you don't think that there is a need to send sex messages. However, this is where you are wrong. Do you remember when you first started dating? You would probably send sexy and interesting messages that you both looked forward to and you would not wait to see each other again and probably act out those fantasies. If you want to bring that spark back into your marriage then you had better consider sexting. Sexting is fun, thrilling, and exciting and by the time you see each other in the evening you are all excited and you know what happens from there. I know it can be hard but just start slowly and build up to sexting and you will be amazed at what it can do for your marriage.

Physical Contact

Expert psychologists say that a touch by someone you love can rekindle a spark inside you, which is why they advise their clients coming in for marriage counseling to touch each other often throughout the day, so their bodies become familiar with each other once again and they become tempted to explore each other further once more. Touching the arm, a light rub on the neck, or a pat on the legs are playful touches that can help you and your spouse bring back intimacy into your relationship. Make sure to do it more often, so your spouse knows you want them to come closer to you. Soon, they will start becoming playful with you as well.

Go on Dates

There was some time in your life when you and your spouse used to go on dates frequently. However, things aren't the same as before, but they can be. By simply doing what you guys did before, you can save your marriage. Make each other feel special by going on dates frequently. Surprise them with a candlelit dinner and then a serene walk by the beach. Treat them to a romantic picnic on the weekend or take them to a local but good bed and breakfast for a romantic day out. Make sure to keep everything romantic and smooth on your date and try not to bring up an upsetting topic or talk about kids, work and other responsibilities. Just be in the moment and enjoy each other's company and you will be amazed at what this can do for you.

Don't Set Limits

Once things start improving between the two of you after practicing the tips outlined in this book, you need to take care of one thing. Never set limits on what time and how many times you guys should spend time together and have sex. Be intimate and do whatever you feel whenever you feel like. Never stop your spouse from coming close to you because it's daytime or because you just did it. Just enjoy each other's company and closeness and celebrate the love you have because setting limits takes away freedom from you and this makes your life monotonous and exhausting.

Also, plan something special for your date nights. You could decorate the room with candles, or put on some romantic music to set up the mood and make your spouse drawn towards you.

Lots of interesting tips, right? Now, it is your job to implement them, so things become smooth and amazing for you and your better half once more.

Chapter 12: Tantric Sex For Marriage

When you begin to follow the path of tantric sex, you begin to find a change in yourself. You find yourself changing how you view yourself and how you view the world. You find yourself looking at relationships that will last a lifetime. Through your journey, you will learn that every man and woman has a certain level of divinity in them. You will start to view sex as a sacred act instead of just a physical act. You will also learn to love deeper and find that you are soaring to different levels of bliss.

You will only have a successful journey when you relieve yourself from any preconceived notions. You should not think of what you need to do and what your lover must do to please you. When you read this chapter, you will be able to identify new ideas about yourself and also embrace new ideas about yourself. You will also learn how to have great sex!

You will learn the basic concepts of tantric sex and identify new exciting ways to life and love. This chapter will be worth it!

The Yin and the Yang: Which is male and which is female?

You must be familiar with the stereotypes that men are from Mars and women are from Venus. This implies that men are assertive and extremely powerful while women are soft and fragile who are only fit for nurturing. There are other stereotypes that men do not show any feelings whatsoever, while women have a plethora of emotion that is ready to unleash itself in a second. It has also been said that women do not take credit for the work that they do, since being outgoing is something only men are familiar with. Over the last few years, there has been a drastic change in the way men and women think.

Tantric sex is a firm follower of the fact that men and women do have opposite characteristics. This is the elementary principle of the Tantra. The eastern theories claim that Yin represents feminism while Yang represents masculinity. But there is no concrete proof that a woman cannot have Yang characteristics or that a man cannot have Yin characteristics. Rather than viewing men and woman as two entities, you should begin to focus on the energies. The Tantra believes in the amalgamation of these two energies.

Shiva and Shakti

The most common image of the Yin and the Yang is the Hindu divine couple Lord Shiva and Goddess Shakti. Lord Shiva represents the entire universe since he is considered the creator and Goddess Shakti represents the root of all energy. The union of the two deities creates a longing in you and every other human being to be treated as a god or a goddess. This is discussed in detail in the following chapters. You will learn to worship your partner as a god or a goddess.

The male energy that is found in Lord Shiva represents ecstasy while the energy in Goddess Shakti represents wisdom. This magical combination is what helps a person attain enlightenment. This perfect couple is always represented in numerous entwined positions – either dancing, or embracing or standing together. There are other positions where Goddess Shakti is wrapped around Lord Shiva with her legs propped around his hips. The dancing position by far is the most sacred since they are able to free their spirit, giving them a chance to attain enlightenment.

Understanding the opposites

You may have made divisions amongst you and your partner. You have to first identify and understand these divisions to strike a balance between the opposite energies. There are quite a few stereotypical characteristics that you may relate to. You will have to identify those characteristics and make note of them. You have to go from one extreme to the next. You should ask your partner to do this too. You will then have to see how you can embrace the extreme characteristics that you and your partner have. You have to identify how you can strike a balance between the polarities that exist between you and your partner. You will have to identify the Yin to your partner's Yang and vice versa.

You might now wonder if it is true that opposites attract. Sit back and think for yourself. You will be able to answer this question on your own. Try analyzing your past relationships. See how you and your partner were different from each other. Identify whether the differences were complemented by each other. This will help you analyze your future relationships as well.

My partner is my beloved
Tantra is not mad love but sacred love. You are honoring your partner and cherishing your partner while making love. You will shower unconditional love on your partner. When you are talking to your partner,

use loving words like 'darling' or 'beloved'. You will find that those little words have aroused feelings of love within your partner. Call your partner with the aforementioned loving words when talking about him or her in public. You might find it terribly strange to do so but you will be sending out a message of love to the person you are speaking to.

The Desire Spectrum
You will find yourself with new views of desire. You may feel a desire every time you think of someone. You may comment on how you want a guy or how hot a girl is when you see them passing. You only feel these desires when you feel incomplete. Since you feel incomplete, you always want another person. You find yourself feeling needy and feeling wanted. But when you do get the person you want, you begin to want something more. You want someone prettier, more interesting and sometimes someone richer. Through tantric sex, you will be able to detach yourself from superficial needs. This will help you create a healthier relationship with your partner.

You feel empowered to say what you want!
When you find yourself empowered, you are able to set boundaries both during sex and in life in general. You

find yourself with a new level of self – esteem. In tantric sex, you OWN your body and your soul. When your partner wants you to enter you, he must ask for your permission. You should not be afraid and have to say yes or no as the situation demands. You have to stop and say that you do not want to be touched in a way that is not comfortable with. You empower your partner when you speak the truth this way. You will be giving your partner the methods to use to please you. You have to be okay with how you are touched and how you feel.

Chapter 13: Teachings of tantric sex

In this chapter we will look at certain teachings of tantra that will help you increase the intimacy; sexual pleasure and it will also help you change your life and relationships for the better. When these teachings are made proper use of then they can also help you take a step closer to enlightenment. Each one of these teachings can be used in two ways, a sexual and a non-sexual way.

Breathe

Remember to breathe. If you have noticed, then you would have realized that a lot of importance has been given to breathing in almost all the teachings that have originated in the East and these teachings can help you attain enlightenment. It is essential that you understand why this is done and the manner in which it is related to Tantra and spiritual development as well.

The answer is quite simple, we all breathe all the time and if we stop breathing for too long it might result in death or becoming unconscious. In this manner, it can be understood that breath is related to our consciousness. Breath can be thought of as energy; every breath we take fills our body with a fresh burst of oxygen and takes away the carbon dioxide. This oxygen is in turn supplied to all the cells in the body. Breath and oxygen can be thought of as fundamental needs of our body. Breathing is not a conscious but an unconscious function. You might not pay attention to whether or not you are breathing, but you never really stop breathing till the day you die. Your life is dependent on something that you don't even do voluntarily.

What would happen if we were to make breathing a conscious effort? All the teachings from the East, including Tantra, make relating a conscious function and this will help transform the way the practitioner of these functions. Like I have stated earlier, breath is energy. And by being able to regulate your breathing, you will be able to regulate the energy generated as well.

You might be able to notice some interesting things if you can focus on not just your own breathing, but also that of your partner while engaged in a sexual activity. It is quite common that while having sex, people engaged in it tend to either hold in their breath for a few moments when they get excited. And then they let out a lot of the air that they were holding on to. When you halt your breathing in such a manner and then let it all out by a jolt, then the energy flowing in your body is likely to be disrupted as well. When you make breathing a conscious act during sex, you will learn how to control the movement of energy instead of just allowing it to flow in the body.

This teaching of tantra is all about breathing in a relaxed manner, take deep breaths, do not stop breathing and don't tighten your lungs. Let the breath flow freely. Only when you do this will the energy flow through your body freely. When your breathing is short or even shallow, this ends up choking the energy in our body.

If you want to achieve a full-body orgasm then it becomes easy when you breathe deeply. Focus on your breathing and allow it to move without any restrictions in your body. Feel the breath filling and then leaving your lungs fully.

Relax

In the same manner, in which shallow breathing can obstruct the flow of energy while participating in sex, the tension in your muscles will also do the same. The muscular tension that you experience during sexual activity is not a conscious one, but an unconscious one. The principle of tantric sex is to make this muscular tension a conscious decision to help you become aware of all the muscles that are being held up. You do require some tension to facilitate the movement if body and for also holding up the body, but that's about it. Muscular tension is not needed everywhere.

If you make the decision of tensing up your muscles a conscious one, you will observe that during sex you tend to tense up some muscles unnecessarily. A man might tense up his muscles even while enjoying oral sex. All he needs to do is lie down on his back and enjoy the ministrations provided to him by his partner; even then he might end up tensing his muscles in his torso and legs. In this case, you would notice that none of this tension is required. Let the energy flow without any restrictions in the body. Focus your attention on not just relaxing your muscles but also on breathing. Enjoy the warmth of the sexual energy that is flowing through your body.

However, it is essential that you understand that relaxation is required of not just your body but your mind as well. Let go of all the expectations, just enjoy the activities you are involved in. bask in the warmth of this energy. Let go of all the unnecessary emotions; don't hold yourself back.

Sounds can help!

Sounds are critical for the movement of energy as well. Some people might not be comfortable or they might even be self-conscious or nervous about the way they sound, but don't take this consideration seriously while considering tantric sex.

Let go of all your inhibitions. Express yourself freely and without any restrictions. Make all those sounds that can express the way you are feeling while engaged in the act. These sounds that you make involuntarily can be referred to as connected sounds. That is, these sounds are connected with the emotions or even sensations that you are experiencing. These sounds will help in the unobstructed flow of energy in your body.

If you are quiet or silent, then the movement of energy becomes difficult. But when you are loud or vocal, then the energy can start moving freely in your body. The more sounds you make, the pleasure quotient you experience will also be more. So, the noise you make is directly proportional to the pleasure you experience. The more connected these sounds are to your emotions and sensations, the more freely and powerfully the energy can move within your body.

If you trying to decipher the sounds associated with each of these emotions and come up blank, don't worry, because these sounds will be generated only while you are experiencing something. Think about all the pleasurable times, it might make you gasp or moan slightly, some experiences might just cause you to intake a sharp breath. All these will contribute to the sounds that you make while engaged in sexual intercourse. Everything that you feel has a sound. The sound produced need not be coherent, it is just about expressing your emotions in a vocal manner.

While having sex, there might be some experiences that make you feel ecstatic and this will be expressed in the sounds you make. But on the other hand, there might be some experiences that might be unpleasant or painful. Do not hold back on these sensations, if something seems painful, and then make the sound that you are in pain. This will help in letting your partner know that you are in pain. It is not just about being vocal, but you can be verbal as well. Verbal means making use of words to express what you are feeling whereas vocal means the making use of sounds to communicate the same. You have the liberty to say what you are feeling, if you feel that something is unpleasant or painful, express it. If you feel that something is pleasurable or just perfect express that as well. Do not hold back your emotions. When you express yourself through sounds, the energy tends to move faster than while expressing through words.

You can consider the example of a toddler who has just acquired speech. At this age, they communicate their feelings through the sounds they make. Think about a child throwing a tantrum, the gamut of angry sounds they make can help the parent understand that the child is cranky and requires something. All you hear would be a jumble of sounds and hardly any words. Even if words were present, the words would be to the point like a loud "No". Toddlers are capable of expressing their emotions loudly, whether be it their laughter or the wails of their sadness. This is how they express their emotions.

And in the same manner, let go of your inhibitions. Make sounds that you want to, it doesn't matter what they sound like either to you or your partner, because these sounds are capable of expressing what you are experiencing at a particular moment. The more you keep doing this, the deeper and connected your sexual activity will be and the result will also be much better.

It is really important that I stress the importance of this point. Of all the principles of tantra, this seems to be the one that a lot of people struggle with. Let go of your inhibitions and express yourself freely.

Eye contact is essential

This might sound pretty basic and obvious to some extent. But it really does help make your sexual experience more pleasurable, enjoyable and intense. Looking at your partner while engaged in any sexual act will definitely make the experience more intense. When I say eye contact, I don't mean that you should stare wistfully into the eyes of your partner. Move over the longing look a love-struck puppy has in its eyes, we are talking about some serious X-rated gazing, so get ready for it. This way will definitely help you attain some extra intimacy. For getting started you and your partner can find a comfortable spot to sit so that you both will be able to look into each other's eyes. Take a moment to gather your concentration; usually, a deep breath will do the trick. Once you feel that you are ready, you can open your eyes and gaze into those of your partner. Allow your partner the access to see you, your true self, and in the same manner, you can gaze at them. This might feel a little stupid initially, but trust me when I say that this little trick is extremely effective. And this trick provides you the liberty to incorporate it whenever you want to.

Allow yourself to communicate through your eyes and not just your genitals. You can let your eyes wander over each other's body. Let your partner see the lust in your eyes and the wanton abandonment. Nothing would be a better turn on than knowing that your partner desires you and needs you. In the manner that sounds and touch can communicate, in the same way, you can communicate a lot more by making use of just your eyes alone. This will help you both communicate with each other in an earnest manner.

Pay attention

Energy flows where the attention goes, is a popular saying in the tantric circles. You will have to concentrate on how and where you want the energy to flow. If you are looking to achieve a full-body orgasm, then you will need to focus on your entire body. You will have to pay some attention to feeling those highly sexualized feelings in all your cells as well. A woman who wants to achieve a splendid vaginal orgasm will have to concentrate her attention to deep within herself and pry out all the sexual sensations hiding within. You can make use of the breathing technique and also of muscle relaxation, as well as eye contact coupled with sound to focus your attention and draw out your energy to the spot where you want it to go to. You can choose to focus only on your genitals the place where the sexual energy is stored.

The philosophy of tantra suggests that an individual should let the sexual energy spread all through the body instead of confining it to just one area. To facilitate the energy to move from the genitals and spread through all the different cells. This energy can be used to help revitalize the body or for any other sexual purpose. The energy flow will be where your attention is. So concentrate on that while engaging in sex.

Always be present

The underlying principle of all the teachings is to be present. Present does not just imply being physically present, but mentally present as well. Be present in the moment. Do not wander off to your dreamland or fantasize about anything else. Try to be in the moment with your partner. Be present in what is happening.

Often it so happens that people end up zoning off to their fantasy world while engaged in sex. They close their eyes and drift to their fantasy realms instead of being present in the lovemaking. Sometimes men also do this on purpose. They can think about something completely non sexual to postpone their ejaculation.

This is thought of as being unnecessary in tantra or anything associated to energy work. If you are present, you will be able to endure more of what is happening around you. Only when you are fully aware of what is happening around you will you be able to experience the moment to the fullest. Energy goes where the attention does, and if your attention is fixated on something entirely different, then even your energy will follow suit. Focus your energy on yourself and your lover. Try to be in the moment; do not lose focus of that. And when this happens the potential of seeking greater pleasure will be diminished.

These principles will surely help you to have a better sexual experience when implemented.

Chapter 14: Understand the Challenges Created by Social Messages

These social messages and myths create an array of challenges in both women's and men's sexuality and inhibit people's ability to form satisfying and fulfilling sexual and emotional connections. As a result of these harmful myths and damaging social messages, many relationships end up full of misunderstanding, hurt, and resentment. Instead of seeing these differences and the problems they cause as a result of socialization, people often take them personally or judge their partner inadequate. These differences have negative outcomes for women, men, and couples, and they lead to low sexual desire and dysfunction for women, midlife crisis and dysfunction for men, sexless or low-sex relationships, and emotional disconnection.

Challenges for Women

Distractibility During Sex
Social messages cause women to be distanced from their sexuality and much more easily distracted from their sexual feelings than men are. They are worried

about whether or not it is okay to have sex or are self-conscious about their bodies. Thus it becomes easy for little interruptions to cause women's arousal to drop suddenly. Intrusive thoughts about responsibilities can come in and ruin the mood as well.

Loss of Sexual Interest as a Mom

The image of a good mother is that she is pure, giving, and sexless. Women are supposed to live up to the social ideal of being a perfect caregiver, focused completely on her children. This image makes mothers feel like their needs are selfish, that sex or any other sensual, self-caring pursuits should be suppressed. We've heard so many women say that, when they became mothers, they didn't feel right doing all of the "naughty" sexual activities they once did. They stopped having many of the experiences that used to make them most aroused.

Low Sexual Desire

Many people try to figure out if women's lower desire is socially or biologically determined; we believe it is likely a bit of both. Because of hormonal differences, women have a somewhat lower sex drive; however, as we have explained, social messages also make it hard for women to connect to their sexual selves and cultivate their desire. Women have very high and usually unattained potential for pleasure: they generally experience more full-body sensation than men and can have varied and multiple orgasms. If your partnership has a woman in it, we want to help you move beyond the harmful social messages so that she can experience her full erotic potential.

Challenges for Men

Midlife Crisis

Social messages are often what lead to men's midlife crisis. When we think of midlife crisis, what often comes to mind is a fortysomething man in a shiny red hot rod running off with some younger woman to find himself. Popular representations of this phenomenon paint this man as childish and selfish. The movie fantasy is generally that he wises up, realizes the error of his ways, repents, and returns to his wife and family. This popular depiction misses the point in many ways: it fails to address the underlying emotional, physiological, and societal reasons for this phenomenon. Men's bodies experience an abrupt and significant change in ability near age forty. As men are noticing their own physical decline, many are also seeing their fathers get old or die, which leads them to wonder whether they will get to live their lives the way they want to before they themselves die. The definitions of "good husband" and "good father" rarely leave space for men to continue doing the things they love to do in life without being deemed selfish and uncaring.

Sexual Dysfunction

Men may experience a psychological shutdown to sex because it feels terrible that their partner keeps rejecting their sexual advances. They don't want to push their sexual desires on their partner and are tired of feeling rejected so they stop getting erections. In addition, there is so much pressure on men to be sexual and ready for every sexual invitation that they aren't allowed the build-up they need to stay connected to their partner during sex. Instead, they worry about their performance. Many men experience anxiety and performance issues such as erectile dysfunction, early ejaculation, and delayed ejaculation. In these cases, we think sexual dysfunction is a response to a dysfunctional situation. If a man feels rejected or pushed to perform on command, his penis begins to rebel, as if to say, "I don't like this treatment" or "You can't make me do that." The fact that his penis is saying "no" to things that he doesn't want means it's time to take a look at the situation and see if there is something that needs to change in the relationship, not in him.

Challenges for Couples

Sexless Relationship/Marriage

Many couples come to us because they find themselves in sexless marriages. These marriages might be wonderful in every other way, with plenty of love, companionship, commitment, and cooperation, but one or both partners feel no sexual attraction or desire for the other. This can be a result of the different social messages they received. Sexless marriage can also be a result of partners having different desires (see "Hottest Sexual Movies" below) and not knowing how to communicate the differences. It may also simply be that one or both of them has lost attraction for the other.

As a result of social messages, women experience low desire and men feel inadequate and overwhelmed with sexual urges. This is not always the case, as a man can be very repressed around his sexuality and his partner more open due to an accepting sexual socialization. In general, however, the one who wants sex more will try to initiate and get rebuffed repeatedly. Eventually, that person will begin to feel rejected and undesirable, give up, and stop trying.

There is nothing inherently wrong with having a sexless marriage, provided that you are honest with each other and agree that it is what you want. If either or both of you want sex, then you may be able to learn how to reconnect with each other sexually. This section will help you find the energy, playfulness, and technique to meet each other's sexual needs. Alternatively, you may have to face your disappointment about your loss of desire and attraction and figure out how you will handle it. Reading about disappointment in Part 2 of this book can be helpful.

Emotional Distance

Men's and women's differing socialization can lead to a relationship that lacks intimacy, empathy, and connection. It is much easier to have empathy for someone when you can understand and relate to their feelings, fears, and desires. Because women's sexuality is repressed and men's emotionality is repressed, relationships can be full of emotional misunderstanding. In relationships, women often feel overly emotional or "too much," and men get labeled as emotionally unavailable. Because they are repressed and their expression is usually less overt, men's emotions can end up being left out.

Affairs

The emotional distance and sexless relationships that result from all of this misunderstanding often lead to affairs. One partner feels like some of their deep sexual or emotional needs are not being fulfilled. Often they still love their partner and try to get those needs met elsewhere without breaking up their relationship or family.

One Couple's Plight Through the Lens of Social Messages

Mandy and Phillip came to us seven years into their marriage. Phillip dragged Mandy into the session because he wanted to have a better sexual connection with her. He shared that he had felt so much closer to Mandy when they had an active sex life, and he missed their connection. Mandy had not wanted to come because she thought sex was the only thing Phillip wanted from her. She also said that sex was not pleasurable and was sometimes painful for her. She felt like Phillip just wanted to use her and that he didn't care about her or their children. They both had very time-consuming careers, and Mandy felt that any spare time they had should be focused on their co-parenting. Phillip felt that they both gave a lot of time and energy to being parents, and he missed the wild woman he'd married.

They spoke of each other in very judgmental terms. Phillip described Mandy as "frigid," while Mandy said Phillip had a "one-track mind" and didn't care about anything but sex. Mandy did not want Phillip to touch her in any way, because she was suspicious that any time Phillip tried to physically connect with her it was only because he was trying to get sex. They spent the entire session blaming and shaming each other for how they'd ended up, which was so clearly shaped by the social messages they'd been given.

It took them three years to come back for a second session, and by then they were on the verge of divorce. Mandy had caught Phillip cheating, and they were both overwrought. Phillip shared, "I tried everything to get Mandy to see that I was invested in our family and the children, but I just started to feel like I was dead inside, like there was nothing left that made me want to get out of bed anymore. I couldn't even get it up to masturbate." Mandy added, "I didn't realize how depressed Phillip was, but I can't believe he went outside the marriage and betrayed me like that! I still can't believe that sex is more important than anything else to him, even his family."

It took Mandy and Phillip months to begin to see how badly they had missed and misunderstood each other. Because Mandy had been taught that sex was dirty and unimportant, she didn't realize it was one of the main ways that Phillip felt accepted and emotionally connected to her. Phillip realized that he had been judging Mandy harshly, calling her frigid without realizing how she was struggling to be herself in the midst of the pressure to be a good girl, a good wife, and a good co-worker. As they started to see that they were both longing for deep connection as well as self-expression, they began to support each other and forgive each other for all the misperceptions and judgments. We were sorry to see that it had to get to this point of devastation before they were willing to really face each other's needs and feelings.

Chapter 15: Romance After The Kids

Children are wonderful little human beings, and as your family grows, you will most often find that your relationship with your spouse can suffer. It's not the fault of the kids though. They just happen to take up a lot of your time, and life as you knew it is changed. Now, whenever you want to go somewhere you have to plan ahead, so any spontaneity that you once enjoyed with your spouse has been thrown out the window. Children create more mess; therefore your daily chores multiply significantly. They are also very demanding of your attention, so you end up spending less time with your husband or wife, and have what seems to be no time to yourself at all. But, having children doesn't mean that the romance has to die between couples. You just need to have a plan in action to ensure you still get the time you need to have some adult time.

Update Each Other Every Week

Parents can often feel like passing ships – one is often running out the door just as one is running in. With work schedules and kids to take care of, there's little time to go round. This is particularly true when your children are very young, as they have no independence skills, so they have to rely on their parents entirely. A trap couples often fall into is one of moaning about the negatives that have taken place during the week. To prevent this from happening, set aside some time (even if it's just half an hour) each week where you and your spouse can sit down and update each other about the week that has just passed. Make an effort to share something positive that has happened, or a funny story about something the kids have done that the other might not be aware of. Then, talk about a negative event that occurred. Try and keep the positive and negative comments even, so if you have 3 positives, only talk about 3 negatives. This little bit of time you share with each other every week can make a lot of difference towards keeping up communication between you. It will also help you reconnect with your spouse after such a hectic week.

Sharing the Parenting

Sometimes, depending on work requirements, one parent may feel that they are taking on the full job of taking care of the kids and the house. Try and create a schedule so both parents are involved in the childcare, and both have some time out. Having time to destress can change your mood and how you interact with your spouse and your children, and this makes for a happier household. When the burden of raising children is shared, even if it's not entirely equal, both parents will feel as though they are cooperating with each other and working together. The reason this can enhance the romance in your marriage is because if you are both more relaxed, and one doesn't feel as though they are doing more than the other, then you both will feel supported and appreciate your partner more.

Finding Time for Intimacy

Finding the time to be intimate with your spouse can be extremely difficult, especially when the children are babies or toddlers. Half of them won't sleep during the night, so you may be up and down all night settling your child. It's very hard to relax and feel romantic if you constantly have one ear out listening for the sounds of a crying baby. Then, of course, there is the exhaustion, especially during the baby years. Raising and taking care of a baby takes a lot of energy, and in this modern world, many mothers have to return to work early on to help support the family. So, you have work during the day, chores at night, and child-caring duties to take care of before you can even think about slipping into bed. Then you can almost guarantee that as soon as you start something in the bedroom, the little one will have a screaming fit, or a nightmare. Wait till they're older and they burst into the room unannounced! It's no wonder that intimacy and romance often falls to the wayside once children come along. So how on earth do you find the time? Well, it's definitely no easy task, but with a bit of planning and by becoming opportunists, it can be done. In the first instance, send baby to grandma's for the night. A night to yourselves can be hugely rewarding. If that's not possible, then you need to be ready for any opportunity that may arise. If your baby is in the early phases of sleep, take the chance. If your baby wakes up and you are in the middle of an intimate moment, remember that it doesn't hurt to let them cry for a few minutes. Learn to switch off temporarily from the crying sounds. This isn't easy for many people, especially mothers, but it can become a necessity. You need to find time for intimacy on a regular basis, or you may end up in a relationship where intimacy has completely gone.

Get Yourselves a Babysitter

For any chance at romance after children, you need to find yourselves a really good babysitter that you can trust. This could be a relative that takes your child for the night or someone who comes into your home and watches your child for you. If you have to hire a babysitter it may cost you a little money, but the time you get to spend alone with each other will be well worth it. Get out of the house, away from all the chaos, and just enjoy spending time with your spouse. Don't be tempted to ring the babysitter every 5 minutes to check up on them either. If you hire someone you trust, you have nothing to worry about. Make sure you hire them for more than an hour or two as well. It will take you a while to wind down and relax, so there's no point going out for an hour then coming back. For some couples, it is more helpful if they book a night at a motel or hotel. Completely getting away can really help couples relax and get in the mood for romance and intimacy. Far better than being at home surrounded by laundry, dishes, toys, and diapers.

Pay More Attention To Your Spouse

When they are little, and in some cases when they are older, children have no manners when it comes to interrupting adults. You may be on the phone and have a toddler pulling on your sleeve the whole time demanding your undivided attention. Or as a couple, you may be having a conversation and all you can hear next to you is mum...mum...mum...This is extremely frustrating, for the mother that is being harassed and the father that is trying to have a conversation. At first, this will seem very difficult to do, but you must learn how to ignore your child. Temporarily of course! Children are very distracting and your concentration levels drop significantly when being interrupted, so the sooner you can teach them not to do it the better. If the child absolutely demands your attention right now and you can't even listen to your spouse, then explain to your spouse that you will just sort the child out then get straight back to the conversation. As your child gets a little older, there are other things you can do to prevent interruptions. If as a couple you like to spend time after dinner talking over coffee or a glass of wine, explain to the child that every night after dinner they are to go and play for 30 minutes. Tell them you will come and get them when the time is up, or give them an electronic timer so they can see the minutes ticking down. This half an hour gives you the opportunity to talk to each other and reconnect.

Appreciation, Admiration and Affection

These three words are ones you need to ingrain in your mind for future reference. No matter how busy or how bad a day you have had, remember to show each other some appreciation, admiration and affection. Tell your spouse how you appreciate the help they have given you that day, or because they have stepped in and taken over one of the chores when they got home. Let your partner know you admire how they handled a particular situation involving the children. It could be for dealing with a sick child, or having to reprimand the child. And always show your partner some form of affection every single day. It could be a gentle touch, a kiss, a love note, or telling your partner they look nice today. Every person is looking for these 3 things from someone; it's what we all crave. Someone to show that they care and that they are thankful for our support. Making your spouse feel worthwhile will increase their self-esteem, and romance will be rekindled.

Chapter 16: Improving Intimacy

People often express their desire to love and be loved, to be accepted and known for who we are, to be in a safe relationship, hoping to share out failings and dreams. Is it intimacy that people truly want?

There are so many times when people will use the term intimate in a completely physical context. People can call a couple intimate to express the fact that they have a sexual relationship. But the truth is that this is a narrow and misleading use of the word because there are different types of intimacy:

- Emotional
- Sexual
- Experiential
- Intellectual

Sexual Intimacy

There are times when everybody hungers for a sexual connection, and this is a physical longing. We may not only yearn for intercourse, but also just the presence and touch of another person with their own sensual splendor; the textures, sounds, scents, tastes, and the visual aspects also play a part.

During sex, barriers are lowered, and another person is allowed to your private personal space. This type of intimacy involves some trust and vulnerability. There will be times when everybody wants sex and not lovemaking. This can happen without any attachments, with a bit of affection, or between friends. If you pay attention, you can understand the little nuances of sharing your body and not your heart.

Emotional Intimacy

Sometimes we are interested in finding an emotional connection; accepting yourself, loving yourself, sharing happiness and tough times. People crave comfort, closeness, and trust. People want to have a special connection with a person on a deep emotional level.

This type of intimacy doesn't need physical affection, though for some it can be enhanced by holding hands or a kiss on the cheek.

Two people can be married for years, and they never reach emotional intimacy; remember that intimacy is not a destination but an experience or a group of feelings. Communication is important when it comes to emotional intimacy, but people tend to communicate about life superficially.

People also use activities, humor, and sarcasm to fill up the time they spend together. Whether intentional or not, people tend to "deflect and protect" so that they can avoid transparency and vulnerability that people need in order to thrive as a couple.

The vulnerability that is needed for emotional intimacy produces anxiety for many people. A good way to help get rid of this anxiety is to allow plenty of time to pass so that you can establish trust. The vulnerability can still prove to be tough especially if you're out of practice.

While many people view sex as a relationship glue from where intimacy and communication will flow, others see emotional intimacy as a prerequisite to a good sex life. So, what if this vulnerability isn't going to happen? What if your significant other isn't willing, or can't communicate on a deep and personal way? Even if you have amazing sex, will an unsatisfying amount of emotional intimacy leave you wanting more?

Everybody Experiences Intimacy Differently
Sexual and emotional intimacy tends to be tricky because there are no absolutes. What everybody needs when it comes to intimacy can vary. The way one person deeply shares will be different than the next.

In the same way, our comfort with emotional and sexual intimacy is going to change some over time and evolve with the relationship we're in and the circumstances. Take this, for example, a woman who was married for 20 years is now divorced. To say the very least, the mere thought of stripping off in front of a new lover may cause anxiety, so she could choose to establish a mutual emotional intimacy foundation before any sexual activity. Or she could go the route of detachment with a hookup instead of putting her heart out there.

There are some people that are found with keeping sex at arm's length from their emotions, which makes their lives a lot less complicated. There are single mothers out there that explicitly operate like this, given that having to deal with their ex, raising their kids, and hold down a job is an emotional overload.

There are others that need a convergence of sexuality with connection, agreement, transparency, and trust, which is the definition of emotional intimacy. This all depends on communication and time.

But passion isn't decided through emotional intimacy, just like emotional intimacy doesn't have to have any physical contact. Love is able to happen at an emotional remove or even a sexual remove for that matter. Connection, sex, love: these are what make up the best mix of satisfaction and comfortableness for both people in a relationship.

How to Deepen Your Sexual Connection

If you're interested in bringing more intimacy into your sex life with your partner, instead of it just being sex, here are five things that can help deepen that intimacy.

1. Realize the importance of creating an intimate friendship with your significant other

A lot of people tend to focus too much on the technique during sex. However, your relationship with your partner is a lot more important for feelings of intimacy. The sense of safety, mutual trust, and emotional connection in your relationship is needed in order to bring the intimacy to your sexual desires. Basically, you should work up to the feeling that you are living with somebody that you crave so much, that makes the actual sex even more pleasurable.

2. Become deeply connected with your body

All the stresses of every day like can keep many of us from being able to keep a thorough and consistent self-care routine. As a result, many will devote only a small amount of time enjoying, embracing, and exploring our own bodies. The effects of stress will often trickle into the sex life. When a person doesn't have an intimate and comfortable relationship with their self, it's almost impossible to create an intimate and comfortable sexual relationship with their partner. If you make a space to love, feel, and explore your own body, you will be able to communicate better about what you want, what makes you feel fulfilled, and what you crave.

3. Speak up

A big reason as to why sex will begin to feel like a routine, and a lot less passionate, is because there isn't enough communication. You may see it as overreacting if you voice how upset you were when your partner gave your friend flirty eyes. It would seem unnecessary to speak about how upset you were when your partner didn't ask your opinion when planning your date. But look at it this way: when you suppress your emotion, it isn't going to go away, it will show up again somewhere else.

A way that it will show up is through suppressed intimacy, any form of intimacy. If you can shorten the time between when you were upset about letting that person know, the lower your resentment levels will be. Less negativity means you will have a better willingness to receive and give in different ways, especially with sex.

4. Embrace the dark, light, and everything in between

It's easy for couples to fall into sexual monotony, and it typically coexists with safety. But if you can widen your expressiveness range, it can open the door to a deeper spiritual connection, and this typically means getting out of your safety zone. You may be worried about bringing up something that is "bad," but stepping into that area could be what you need. During sex, it could mean letting your partner take you with more abandon and strength.

5. Surrender to what happens

A lot of the disconnection during sex can come from the pressure of achieving something. This could mean having an orgasm, trying to look good, or being seen as good in bed. It will distract you from the beauty and sacredness of the moment. Maybe you should look at the outcome as experiencing this moment with your partner. If you weren't pressured into reaching a milestone while being intimate, how deeper could your relationship go, and surrender to your partner?

Chapter 17: More Intimacy in 7 Days

You just have to mesmerize your partner with mind-blowing sex to really keep them and have deep bonding with them. Just a quickie in the bathtub or some dry kisses before rolling over will not cut it. You need to satisfy your partner in some well-planned steamy sex session that will leave them always horny anytime they are around you, in fact, they can't literally get their hands off you. Having a bomb ass sex with your partner will make you the woman feeling sexier while the man will have a deep connection with you. it is good to make sex a lot more fun that will drive your partner crazy, use sultry sex positions that will make them explode in ecstasy and will help remind him or her always why you are in a relationship with your them

It is pertinent you turn to sex positions that will strengthen or build the deep connection you need with your partner. .whether you are trying to rekindle the flames of a real love or trying to foster a more profound link with someone new, you need to try out the below hot sex positions that will enable you both to always be in the mood for intense orgasmic sex session filled with fire and deep connection. This will aid your partner fall in love with you all over again.

- Side by side position

You can get your love flames burning very high for deep connection using this sex position. This sex position will leave you both gasping for breathe after the hot sex session and it will foster deep connection because of eye contact and physical closeness it afford the partners during the sex session. With this sizzling position, you and your partner will be delving into a new world of pleasure because the position offers the man the opportunity to get explicit access to your woman's G-spot while pleasuring himself too. This position also promotes deep bonding and makes the woman sexier through the eyes gazing by the partners, kissing is done effortlessly, and there is ease of communication too since the partners can see one another's responses to stimulation. This sex position begins with the man and woman lying side by side by each other; the man draped his leg over the woman's hip so that he can pull the woman's vagina deeper into him. The woman can sometimes have her knees bent up to her breasts for a deeper penetration. To heighten the sexual heat the man should ask the woman to part her thigh a bit, the man would then use his cock to rub her clitoris and allow her scream in excitement for a while before penetrating deeply and thrusting forth and back again still both climax.

- Spooning position

This is a perfect sex position that will make partners scream off their lungs in ecstasy as the pleasure one another, this position is both a sexual position and a cuddling technique, so one can imagine the orgasmic thrills partners will enjoy when using this hot sex position. This sex position will leave the woman feeling sexier and having a strong connection with her partner. The position is a rear-entry position which is like the doggy style position and it is ideal for partners that need a deeper and more pleasurable sensation, it a great position since it allows partners to work through the action of sex together. Spooning sex position puts less strain on the muscles which makes the couple last for long while making love. This sex position has the man lying on his side while the woman lies in front of the man facing away, so this means that the woman will be in the inner spoon position while the man will be in the outer spoon position preparing for the entry penetration. The man enters her from behind; the man can add more sensation by grabbing and fondling with her breast from behind, stimulating her clitoris and finally going anal with her before climaxing.

- Doggy style

A psychosexual therapist based in Palo Alto, California, said that this sex position gives partners orgasmic thrills especially the women deep penetration that leads to immense pleasure and can help the partner have some deep connection after the steamy sex session. So if you need a sex position that will give your partner the adrenaline rush and keep sexual flames burning in the relationship while also keeping you the woman sexier and create deep connection for you both in the relationship, then using the doggy style will just be it. The doggy sex position is pretty easy the woman lies on her stomach with her butt in the air, maybe with a pillow under her pelvis for extra support, the man stands behind her to penetrate from behind but before then he can stimulate the clitoris to bliss with a vibrator. The man can make the woman scream more by introducing anal sex and cap it up with vagina sex but must apply plenty of lube and continue deep thrusting still the both erupt in multiple orgasms.

- The chair sex position

You can't get it wrong with this naughty sex position especially when it comes to sex making that will create deep bonding because of the close body contact involved with this position. The position gets the man all excited since he will be the one sitting and taking in all erotic view of the entire woman's body. The woman on the other hand who is on top of the man will be having it easier with the stimulation of her clitoral and G-spot with this position. The good thing about this position is that it enables the partners to find the right spots to stimulate and the intensity and speed can build up from there. The position will help the partners ditch the bed for a chair so using the chair than a bed will add some zing to the already sizzling sex position. So you can check out the chair position because it will not only add romp to your sex session but foster deep connection and intimacy with your partner. This sex position start with the man sitting upright on the chair and the woman sitting on the man but backing him, The man can start with foreplay like fondling, fingering and stimulating the clitoris and massaging each other bodies, then the woman gently now direct the erect cock to her vagina and lean forward so that she can have the ease of deep penetration while moving her hips up and down in circles which could be backward or forward. To heighten the sexual pleasure the woman can turn around to stimulate all the erogenous zones with her hands and mouth and this will help put fire on both bodies, drawing you both together to create a better connection that can't be denied. The man can take over now and ride the woman to stupor with some deep thrusting.

- Woman on top sex position

Woman on top sex position is a build up on the missionary sex position where the woman is on top. This sex position is classic for partners that really want to connect emotionally with one another through good sex. Apart from the hot sex romp, this sex position offers partners it also offers deep connection through direct eye contact, sexy sounds and sensual touches and there is much more control of deep penetration too with this sex position. This sex position according to Zoldbrod will help the woman on top have clitoral stimulation which will make her reach multiple orgasms in the course of the sex session. This sex position can be started with the man lying on his back while the woman is comfortably on top, the woman grabs the man's penis and give it a huge blowjob to stretch the erection and to build up sensation before directing it to her vagina to insert, the woman leans her body forward and her hand beside or on the man head on the bed for support. The woman will then use her hips to rock back and forth or side by side till she can find the angle that let her rub her clitoris against the man's lower abdomen or pubic bone. This will make the man be practically caged inside the woman as she brings herself almost to climax. She can also engage the man's view by throwing her booty in his face while riding him hard forth and back. The man can be spanking the woman butt and responding to the rhythm of the ride still both climax.

- The lotus sex position

The lotus sex position is called the deep connection sex position because it provides face to face intimacy that can boost deep connection with a partner while making love. This sex position elicit excitement and erotic feelings, with this sex position the bodies are touching entirely and the partner's faces are close enough to have some fun together, there's intense eye contact, whispers, naughty talks and kisses are sure to follow with this sex position. If you need to feel sexier and have a deep connection with your partner then you need to try out the lotus sex position, you will sure have all that you had needed. Start this sex position with the woman sitting with her legs loosely crossed, while the man sits on top of the woman facing her and with his legs wrapped around the woman's back. The man penetrates the woman that way and focus now on moving up and down with slow sensual movement to build sexual thrills gradually. The woman can as well be grinding and rocking to the man rhythm, to build more orgasmic sensation the woman should put her arms under the man's arm and reach to grab his shoulders; this will make room for the woman to pull herself up and down on the man while intensely grinding and rocking him. There should be intermittent kissing, smooching, fondling, naughty talks etc in between. The man can heighten the pleasure to achieve back-arching, toe-curling screaming orgasm by thrusting and grinding deeply.

- Hold me sex position

Hold me a sex position can give partner spine-tingling pleasure while facilitating emotional intimacy and deep connection. This sex position will always leave the partner asking for more as the pleasure one another and also help to build the deepest connection because this sex position offers the opportunity of partners having eye contact, caressing and kissing themselves during the course of this sensational sex session. Hold me a sex position can be done anywhere so you can skip the bedroom and your usual routine with this sex position. This sex position will need the man standing upright and the woman first going on her knees to give the man a good suck on his cock, then she now jump on the man and the man need to hold the woman into his arms and the woman should wrap her legs around the man's waist and her arms should be around his neck. This is a typical sex position to promote body contact and connection as the partners come face to face with one another. Before penetrating the woman, the man can finger and stimulate her clit, kiss and suck away, then penetrate the woman now and grab her booty and push it forward so that he can have deep penetration. The woman can as well respond to the rhythm by pushing herself forth and back and to heighten the pleasure the man can place the woman's back against a wall for support and then thrust deeply till they both explode in multiple orgasms.

- Hands-free sex position

This is one sex position that apart from setting partners bodies on fire also connects them passionately when used. The outstanding feature of this sex position is that the sex position enables the partner's hands to be free for more arousal touches. Making love and have a good amount of fingering and erotic touches help ignite swirling sexual feelings and this can bring about massive excitement and thrills for the partners, such that a remembrance of lovemaking by the partner is fascinating and this will help keep them very close and deep into one another. This sex position promotes face to face contact for the partners which will enable them to smile at one another while also having very close eye contact too. Sex position of this nature can make partners be very emotional and want to always be in another arm. This sex has the man sit on a chair while the woman is astride facing him{ that is her legs wide apart on each side of the man's leg} and the woman's feet should be on the floor. This position will enable the man to face the woman, the same with the woman too. With them facing one another they can begin the lovemaking with foreplay, like the man giving the woman some tantalizing kisses, whispers into her ears, cuddle, fondle with the breast before penetrating. If the woman needs more intense pleasure she can be lifting her butt a bit higher while the man is thrusting and this can also help the man to have a deeper thrusting. The free hands they have because of this sex position can be used to rub, tingle and finger other erogenous spots of the body. The whole body feels thrilling sensation and the climax will be heavenly.

- Snow angel sex position

If you are looking for a smooth transition sex position away from your comfort sex style that will give mind-blowing orgasm, then this sex position will be perfect for you and your partner. This sex position would not only bring deep connections but will get your partner moaning and screaming in uncontrollable ecstasy. It is one sex position that hitting the G-spot is made easy and easily accessible as well as the man pleasuring himself to stupor. It just needs the woman to be flexible and agile to get this position right. This sex position has the woman lying on her back while the man is on top of her, the woman then draw her thighs into the man's chest and goes further to place her legs over her shoulders. This position will allow the man to bring the woman pelvis off the mattress, so that the tilt of the woman hips will allow the man to penetrate deeply into her with this position the man will have undeniable access to the woman G-spot. Rock the woman forth and back until the both climax with a bang.

- Missionary sex position

If you are looking for a sex position that will offer sexiness and deep connection in the bedroom then you should try out this good old sex position. No matter how old a trick maybe being creative with it will suffice. This is applicable too to this sex position you just have to use the creative angle that is written in this book. This sex position is perfect for boosting deep connection during lovemaking. From a personal view, this position allows the partners to be able to kiss, lock fingers together, and the proximity allows for some erotic talks that would arouse the partners even more. There is more connectedness with this position because partners will be wrapped in each other's arms, leg intertwined and a lot of eye contact and this will make the partners sexier, and lovemaking will be sweeter. This position can be called a man on top or couple facing each other. While the woman is on her back, the man climbs on top and penetrate the woman from there as in the right old fashioned way. You can add a rabbit vibrator to the mix to get the woman screaming and moaning away. The man can finger the woman's clitoris too to heighten the pleasure, then insert his penis again and thrust deeply until they both come in multiple orgasm.

Conclusion

By using the guidelines, we have set out in this book you can go on and experience the joys of an intimate, loving, sexual bond with your other half. Used correctly, these pointers are a powerful aid to achieving complete satisfaction.

By concentrating less on the amount of sex you are having and increasing the quality of sex, this can take pressure off couples. Ignore those annoying couples that are constantly banging on about "doing it" five times a week. That is not the path to satisfaction for everybody and you both need to agree that when you do have sex you are both in a place to make it great rather than concentrating on managing to have sex every other day!

Enjoy all your encounters! Orgasm or not, long hot sweaty session or a brief quickie before you set off for work. Sex between you should always create special memories and make you smile. Think about how you feel about your partner after sex, do you feel closer to them or do you detach completely afterward. Knowing how you should feel and how you actually feel may seem like a no brainer, but when was the last time you asked yourself how sex makes you feel?

Recognize when there is a lull in your sex life and know when to change things up! Follow some of the tips in this book and change your whole attitude to bedtime! Don't let modesty or embarrassment stop you experimenting with all manner of aids.

Be aware that other factors can affect your attitude to sex and learn how to address them. It is fairly obvious that the more care you show your body the more you will benefit from it when you are being intimate. A healthy body leads to healthy sex, right?? Mentally you also have to be in a good place to get the most out of your love life. If you are depressed or have other mental health issues then you need to seek treatment before you can concentrate on the physical side of your relationship.

Above all, if you are happy with your partner the sex will be better, simple, right? By using the tips to help you fall in love with your partner again you will glow with happiness and this will fuel your attraction to each other and lead to infinitely better sex!

www.ingramcontent.com/pod-product-compliance
Lightning Source LLC
Chambersburg PA
CBHW070906080526
44589CB00013B/1200